Occupational Therapy in Sho.

For Churchill Livingstone:

Editorial Director: Mary Law
Project Manager: Valerie Burgess
Project Editor: Dinah Thom
Copy Editor: Sue Beasley
Indexer: Liz Granger
Project Controller: Derek Robertson
Design Direction: Judith Wright
Sales Promotion Executive: Maria O'Connor

Occupational Therapy in Short-term Psychiatry

Edited by

Moya Willson TDipCOT BA MSc
Joint Director, School of Occupational Therapy and Physiotherapy,
University of East Anglia, Norwich

THIRD EDITION

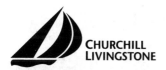

CHURCHILL
LIVINGSTONE

NEW YORK EDINBURGH LONDON MADRID MELBOURNE SAN FRANCISCO
AND TOKYO 1996

CHURCHILL LIVINGSTONE
Medical Division of Pearson Professional Limited

Distributed in the United States of America by Churchill Livingstone Inc.,
650 Avenue of the Americas, New York, N.Y. 10011, and by associated companies,
branches and representatives throughout the world.

First Edition 1984
Second Edition 1988
Third Edition 1996

ISBN 0 443 05396 0

British Library of Cataloguing in Publication Data
A catalogue record for this book is available from the British Library.

Library of Congress Cataloging in Publication Data
A catalogue record for this book is available from the Library of Congress.

The
publisher's
policy is to use
**paper manufactured
from sustainable forests**

Produced through Longman Malaysia, CLP

Contents

Contributors

Gillian Aspinall DipCOT BEd(Hons)
Community Occupational Therapist, Norfolk Mental Health
Care NHS Trust

Kim Atkinson DipCOT MSc
Lecturer in Occupational Therapy, University of East Anglia,
Norwich

Elizabeth Cracknell TDipCOT BSc MA
Former Principal of St Andrew's School of Occupational Therapy,
Northampton

Becky Durant DipCOT DipMH BEd(Hons)
Head Occupational Therapist, Bethel Child and Family Centre,
Mary Chapman House, Norwich

Lynne Howard DipCOT MSc
Lecturer in Occupational Therapy, University of East Anglia,
Norwich

Diana Keable DipCOT BSc(Hons)
Head Occupational Therapist, Mental Health Unit, Northwick
Park Hospital, Watford Road, Harrow

Christine Ravetz DipCOT OTR BA MA
Head of Occupational Therapy Studies, University College of
St Martin, Lancaster

Barbara Steward TDipCOT CertEd BA(Hons) MA
Lecturer in Occupational Therapy, University of East Anglia,
Norwich

Averil M. Stewart TDipCOT FCOT BA
Head of Department of Occupational Therapy, Queen Margaret
College, Edinburgh

Michael Willson BSc MA
Former Consultant in Social Work Management

Moya Willson TDipCOT BA MSc
Joint Director, School of Occupational Therapy and
Physiotherapy, University of East Anglia, Norwich

Preface

Occupational therapy is a fast-moving profession, its hunger for new concepts fuelling its capacity to redefine existing paradigms and describe developing models of practice.

When this book first came out over a decade ago, it made little reference to the models of practice arising from professional literature emanating from the United States and elsewhere. Over the intervening period such models, including, for example, activities therapy and human occupation, have provided a major structural impact upon the way occupational therapy is written about. The impact on the way in which it is practised is less apparent.

A new edition provides an opportunity to place psychiatric practice in the context of currently ascendant models. Happily, it also provides an opportunity to choose not to do so.

In a discussion with a group of students over models of practice, the analogy of the London Underground map emerged. This is an invaluable aid to navigation within the system but bears little resemblance to the reality of what exists above ground. In fact it can distort distances and relationships and can ignore all other interconnecting routes. A particular student was so appalled to realise this for the first time that he swore to traverse the capital only on foot until his mind had grasped the true orientation of its landmarks.

This is not a condemnation of any model, nor yet of the London Underground. This edition will, however, like the previous, concentrate on describing those landmarks which I believe to be important to professional orientation. If students of occupational therapy are familiar with this material then they are well placed to bring a critical appreciation to profession-specific frames of reference and their emergent models.

As before, the book is broken into three major themes, the first addressing the client group. The chapter on mental health remains as a problem-based description since I still believe that this is the most useful introduction, and that diagnostically organised information is easily accessed within general psychiatry texts. Rather than possessing a cornucopia of medicalised labels we need to be sensitive to the multiple distresses of personal 'a-copia'—the broad inability to cope with the demands of living at this turn of the millennium. This theme is taken forward by Averil Stewart in her revised account of stress and vulnerability. This addresses some of the specific difficulties which people encounter and ways in which these may be perceived. An important addition is a new chapter by Gillian Aspinall on the older person in receipt of occupational therapy. The changing proportion of elderly people within the population suggests the need for a specific focus on their experiences.

Chapters 4 to 7 review key concepts which currently influence work in short-term psychiatry. In their choice they represent the interesting tensions between the importance of a theoretical basis and the reality of practising in the current health care climate. Elizabeth Cracknell has extended the essential background on our roots in humanistic psychology to balance the more pragmatic input on cognitive approaches in Chapter 5. Kim Atkinson has provided a new contribution on practice in the community, which is now essential to a book on practice with this client group. Quality, in all aspects of provision and monitoring, has also become a major issue within the practice of every form of professional work. A further new chapter by Lynne Howard addresses this issue.

The last section addresses practice issues and turns attention to a few selected topics. These illustrate some aspects of work with this client group but do not constitute a compendium of all approaches and activities. Diana Keable has contributed a new chapter on the management of anxiety, since this is a particularly significant problem to therapists in the field. Barbara Steward has drawn together the use of a number of expressive media to write a new chapter on the principles and practice of creative therapies. The subject of leisure within this section has been re-addressed by Christine Ravetz. Another new inclusion is a chapter on family therapy by Becky Durant. This is not intended as an instructional guide but as a lively illustration by a practising therapist of the challenges of shifting theory within an area of practice.

I am indebted to all the existing authors who have been willing to contribute to this major revision and have enjoyed the work of the new team who have added their experience and time to bring this new edition into line with current needs. Particular thanks are due to Tracey Hourd for getting the manuscript together, treating blips in my head and on her screen with impartial determination.

Norwich 1996   M. W.

PART 1

The clients

1

Mental health

Moya Willson

INTRODUCTION

Mental illness is a precarious topic. Even a cursory glance at past and present literature reveals it to be the subject of passionate debate. Some of the views held are so opposed that they seem never to penetrate further than problems of definition, and the battlefield becomes one of semantics.

This chapter does not seek to uphold or condemn any particular frame of reference but rather describes the subject and its debate. The emphasis is on the description and disabilities of those who are perceived by others to be 'sick' or 'mad'. An alternative social view of the inability of some people to cope within society is the subject of the next chapter, although it is inevitable that a high degree of overlap occurs.

The word 'madman' is no longer used to describe someone who has a disordered mind. Likewise 'lunatic', 'maniac', 'bedlamite', 'raver' and 'idiot' are terms which have changed their meaning as knowledge and attitudes have claimed greater sophistication. Interestingly, these have all become terms which have a dual purpose of abuse and endearment, depending on the context in which they are used.

If normality or sanity could be defined and understood as a baseline against which abnormality could be measured, then the study of psychiatry would be much easier. As it is, many people now avoid the use of 'normal' or 'sane' in description for fear of being challenged to explain what they mean. Depression, anxiety, antisocial behaviour, addiction, delusion and confusion are all normal features in that they may be represented within the life span of a person who functions adequately, or at least does not appeal for help. These are all symptoms of abnormality when they are present to an incapacitating degree, or when they are recognised in a person who is failing to cope with his life. It may be useful to use the term 'average' rather than 'normal' to describe those who do not come to the attention of professional agencies. Their experience of the world does not cross that line beyond which one does not only worry about oneself but is *worried about* by other people, who ultimately act.

Being outside the average range gives rise to being exceptional. Consider this statement in relation to physical health (Fig. 1.1).

A second very simplified curve shows the same concept applied to mental health (Fig. 1.2). Note that, for convenience, neither diagram includes the bulge of infirmity which is the result of physical accidents.

This seems terribly obvious until one starts wondering why the two vertical lines, which form the boundaries of normal range, are placed where they are. In the diagrams they were placed arbitrarily in order to illustrate a point; in reality they move according to cultural, economic and political pressures. The reasons why these boundary lines move, making the normal range more or less inclusive include the following:

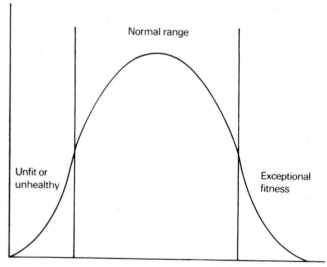

Figure 1.1 A simplified distribution curve related to physical fitness.

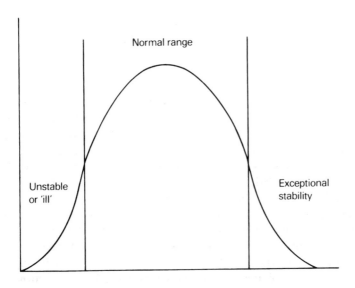

Figure 1.2 The concept illustrated in Figure 1.1 applied to mental stability.

1. *The resources of the community which can be directed towards health or social services.* In parts of the world where survival and physical health are threatened, there is less emphasis on recognising and aiding those who are psychologically disturbed. There also may be less effort made to identify and exploit the strengths of those who are exceptional at the positive end of the scale. On the other hand, wealthy nations or communities can direct more resources to fulfilling the needs of their exceptional members and hence can afford to diagnose more people as being ill in some way. Note that the 'incidence' of any disorder is calculated on the number of times it is diagnosed and may not be a true reflection of the number of people who may be experiencing its effects.

2. *The acceptability of diagnosis and treatment.* Both doctors and their patients are subject to social controls when they seek to define the situation which they are in. On an international level, for example, the diagnosis of schizophrenia is more inclusive in some parts of the world than in others (WHO 1972). Individually, many psychiatrists are becoming more sensitive to the negative effects of diagnostic labelling and are more reluctant to define a patient as not belonging within a normal range of human behaviour and distress. On a social level the negative effects of

stigma may lead to different patterns of self-referral for help. National attitudes and social class are both influential. To give two extremes: in some subcultures a regular appointment with a psychoanalyst or membership of a therapeutic group is almost a mark of sensitive respectability; in others, a disabling degree of emotional distress may only give rise to a belated visit to a general practitioner on the pretext of some related physical complaint.

3. *Reference to opinions or beliefs.* Political ideologies, popular morality or any other doctrines which are allowed to become dogmatic can all be misused. We used to believe that those who held that the earth revolved around the sun were crazy. What attitudes are sometimes held towards those who persist in viewing the theory of evolution as a form of heresy? It is believed in the West that many psychiatric hospitals in other parts of the world are used to curtail the freedom of political dissenters, and this may be so. The more tolerant any society is towards divergence of opinion and belief the less likely it is that minority groups will be defined as abnormal, and subsequently ill-used. It is useful to remember that perceptions of normality in this respect change continually. We no longer imprison women who seek to vote nor commit them to asylums for immorality; we are growing less wary of people who see unidentified flying objects. We are, however, still fairly certain about the invalidity of the claims made by current 'prophets' or 'messiahs'.

4. *The variability of social support.* This is a difficult one and may be a confusing addition, but it does have great significance to those who exist very close to that wobbling vertical line. Individuals who are referred for treatment, either by themselves or others, are often those who are without close friends or relatives or whose family dynamics are a part of the problem. The tendency towards a social structure of nuclear rather than extended families may throw the weak or the peculiar into sharper relief. The frustrations of poverty or unemployment may cement family relationships, may create emotional disorder or may lay bare a previously supported member of the family who can no longer be tolerated. Variations in social support are closely influenced by the previous three points. However, many individuals who share the same apparent degree of incapacity or stress can be identified on different sides of the defining line. The difference between them is the amount of social support which they receive from family or friends.

PSYCHIATRY AND REALITY
Problems of description

Psychiatric disorders are categories which have been invented by psychiatrists. Such categories are usually inclusive of a number of problems and personal circumstances which are frequently found in conjunction with each other. For example, symptoms which include misery, sleep disturbance, preoccupation with bowel function and general retardation, found in conjunction with the menopause and with changes in responsibility, could be recognised by some as being a syndrome. A syndrome is something one has seen before and will probably see again.

It is not, however, always possible to place a whole range of physical, emotional or cognitive experiences along one axis of an imaginary grid, place typical features of personality and biography along the other and identify specific disorders in the way that the mileage between destinations can be found on the chart at the back of a road atlas.

If each psychiatric disorder had a number of unmistakable features, which did not grossly overlap with those belonging to other disorders, then it would be possible to use the study of plants as a parallel. By general examination the family could be established and by closer scrutiny the individual species identified. Some organically based problems, for example both amentia and dementia, will admit such a parallel to a large degree. Other areas of psychiatric concern are either less advanced or more complex than the study of botany. In some cases we can identify the family but are less sure about the species. This might apply to 'schizophrenia'. In other conditions, for example anorexia nervosa, the description of the disorder is precise enough to think that it is a species but there is room for disagreement about the family to which it belongs.

Diseases of the mind

The word 'disease' ought to cause few problems since it has been applied precisely within physical medicine for a very long time. Within psychiatry, however, it provides a useful example of apparent disagreements or confusions which may bother (or stimulate) a student who is new to the subject. Compare the following statements:

Silvano Arieti (Arieti & Bemporad 1978): 'If "disease" means a condition that causes a dysfunction of the organism, irrespective of evidence of cellular pathology and irrespective of the nature of the cause which determined it, we can certainly call depression a disease.'

Christian Scharfetter (1980): 'In psychiatry the medical model of illness can be used only in those mental disorders which are associated with physical illness (especially cerebral disease): acute exogenous reactions, amnestic psychodramas, the dementias, the organic psychoses (brain syndromes).'

Jeff Coulter (1973): 'Why should we think that those phenomena to which we intelligibly refer with the word "disease" should manifest invariant, common properties that we could codify neatly into a list or a definition ... It seems to me that much of the ink that is wasted in constructing definitions of "disease" derives from the attempt in psychopathology to rationalize the use of the medical nosology.'

Incidentally, the word 'nosology' means the study of classification of disorders and the word 'psychiatry', according to the Concise Oxford Dictionary, means 'study and treatment of mental disease'. Now read the personal accounts in Boxes 1.1 and 1.2. They were written by two young people admitted to an acute psychiatric admission unit.

Box 1.1   Young woman of 28

There isn't anything inside me, there isn't anything to feel. I'm not sad because I am not anything and you should not come to me because of the stench ... Because only my bowels are full and I feel that I am rotting. I don't want to eat any more, food will only sustain the badness. You cannot reach me because I have to be alone and I cannot get out because I'm sorry for all the things I've done. Sorry for them, not sorry for me—and you should not be because there is nothing. I have slipped away from myself but my body drags on and anchors my sin.

Having registered their distress, we can continue to 'waste ink' in discussing the general concept of disease or we can state that there is something *wrong* with them in comparison with other people and not worry too much about semantics. Neither course of action would be satisfactory, since one needs to be able to describe a problem with some confidence before attempting to deal with it.

Box 1.2   17-year-old youth

It all started to happen last year one summer and I have had it to this day. That is why I am writing a diary of the action.

1. It first started last summer with worry and strange thoughts. It came to me gradually. It just affected me by making me think that people were putting their worries and problems on to me and leaving their badness on me and on the furniture such as chairs, doors, knives, forks and spoons, money etc. And if I touched them I would get all their worries and problems.

2. Then I thought that people were taking my sight in some way such as if I looked at a book and had turned the page over I thought I had left some of my sight there on the page I was looking at.

3. And if somebody bumped into me or touched me I felt that they were taking my goodness.

4. Or if I was walking along a road and a bus or a car or a person walked past I felt that they were taking part of my body with them. The same thing happened if I walked or ran past a lamp post and I could really feel this strange force taking place.

5. Some time after this sickness I had other thoughts. I felt I was walking on people or on my pet fish. Then one day one of my best fish died. Could this have something to do with what I was thinking? Other things like this happened.

6. Then another thought came. People and places played on my mind and when I thought of a place I felt as if I was going there in spirit and seeing it as it was at that time. Then I thought people were voodooing me and caused things to happen to me and my home.

7. Then I thought everyone was against me. I thought people would rob my thoughts, my sight, my strength and I thought I had a number and if anybody knew that number which is number 12 they would break me, and I thought if I thought of anything at home or anything at all people could see and hear what I was thinking and if I didn't jump up and bless myself they could hear and see what I am thinking. I felt people could rob my ears and if I throw any rubbish away I was throwing my goodness with it and when I walked I felt I was draining out. I stopped this from happening by jumping up and down and blessing myself or going back and touching things, or closing my eyes and getting my sight back from other people. I went to have my eyes tested. They were all right but I still had these things happening to me.

I stopped going out and stopped reading and watching telly. One day when I got round to reading I saw a column about OBE (out of body experience) where people can leave their bodies in spirit.

What a coincidence I thought could this be true, could this be happening to me?

So I am still troubled with these thoughts but I have learned to live with them and I am better now. All the same these things are still on my mind—they could be true.

The way in which different doctors or therapists describe problems is dependent on their previous experience, their education and their beliefs. The next section will therefore summarise several of the different viewpoints which may influence their perceptions of abnormality.

Differing perspectives

In the past, explanations of deviancy were derived from beliefs then held and knowledge then available. Hence the acceptance that it was possible to be possessed by demons or that individuals could be guilty of witchcraft. As an alternative to demonology, early somatogenic theories proposed physical facts which supposedly directed both personality and also aberrant behaviour.

Within current thinking, demonology has given way to the more scientifically based studies of psychology and human relationships. Somatology has matured into a highly sophisticated understanding of how human physiology may influence human behaviour.

The current perspectives, derived from this historical background, are the psychodynamic, the behavioural and learning, the humanistic and the physiological.

The psychodynamic

Also known as the psychoanalytical approach, the concepts derive from theories of personality. Historically the most influential figure in this field is Sigmund Freud. Students of occupational therapy should be aware of the way in which he described mental structures including the roles of the *id*, *ego* and *superego* in directing the personality on both conscious and unconscious levels. Personality theorists place a great deal of emphasis on development and the significance of early trauma or deprivation. Freud describes oral, anal, phallic, latent and genital phases, each of which presents conflicts. The manner in which these conflicts are resolved, or fail to be resolved, influences future pathology in the adult. In Freudian terms, psychological problems are described as fixations and complexes. A fixation, for example anal fixation, denotes a blockage in development which leaves the individual frozen or 'fixed' at a stage in psycho-sexual attraction to either parent figure. Hence the terms 'Oedipus complex' in the male and 'Electra complex' in the female. Freud also described neurotic anxiety which may be 'free-floating', as experienced within phobias, or manifest as 'panic reactions' which are more transient in experience but equally deep-rooted. A failure to resolve developmental conflicts or to deal with anxiety on a conscious level gives rise to defence mechanisms. These include repression, projection, displacement, reaction formation, regression and rationalisation, several of which are described within Chapter 2.

The ideas of Freud, and those who developed and expanded his work and who are known as 'neo-Freudians', form the basis of individual and group psychotherapy today.

Those who adhere to their concepts will seek the explanation for present distress in the biography of the patient and his ability to reveal unconscious material through techniques such as 'free association'. They will translate therapeutic relationships in terms of positive and negative transference and be sensitive to the likelihood of 'projection' when the patient describes relationships, objects or events. Some of these terms may be unfamiliar but they will not be defined or discussed further here since they are well documented. Essentially, it should be understood that personality theorists offer an interpretation which relates to the past, of current experiences of distress or stagnation. Projective techniques, such as the Thematic Apperception and the Rorschach Ink Blot tests are the tools of analysts who work within this frame of reference and are not normally utilised by occupational therapists. Creative activities, using various art forms discussed within Chapter 9, may serve as an adjunct to a psychodynamic approach to treatment. They may assist a patient to identify, and come to terms with, events or emotions which are significant within his own biography and relationships.

Behavioural and learning

Theorists of this persuasion tell us that all behaviour is learnt and hence problems can be described in terms of inappropriate learning or of failure to learn. When problems or anxieties arise, most people adopt strategies which are reasonably successful and which do not, in themselves, give rise to further problems. A tendency to adopt the wrong strategies, or to be socially helpless or in-adequate, can be recognised in many individuals who are described as having psychological disorders. More extreme pieces of behaviour, such as social withdrawal, autism and bizarre or confused speech can be seen as an attempt to escape from personal and social difficulties.

Behaviourists base their descriptions of behaviour, and their attempts to modify it, on the experimental findings of psychologists who have studied learning. Early influences were, of course, Ivan Pavlov who described classical conditioning, and Edward Thorndyke, followed by Frederick Skinner who laid down the foundations of operant conditioning. An appreciation of the types of learning involved in classical conditioning enabled clinicians to develop methods such as desensitisation and aversion in order to change the response made by an individual to a given set of stimuli. Strategies arising from operant conditioning, such as token economy and biofeedback, are used to elicit behaviour from a subject in order to gain a desired response.

More recently, learning theorists have become interested in the social context in which learning takes place. Modelling, as a teaching technique, has emerged from experimental work which demonstrates that watching someone else perform a task, or fulfil a social role, enables the observer to acquire complex patterns of behaviour before active involvement has taken place. Children, of course, learn much of their repertoire of social behaviour in this way. It should be remembered that it is not just observable behaviour which is subject to imitative learning. Attitudes and anxieties can be conveyed from one 'generation' to another by the omission or discouragement of discussion and activity. There is, for example, little opportunity within western society to witness adult sexual behaviour. However, the conditioned emotional responses of parents to sexual stimuli appear to be transmitted to their children. A study of aggressive and inhibited boys (Bandura 1960) indicated that parents who were anxious about sex tended to have sons who experienced guilt in relation to sex and who had difficulty in establishing close, affectionate friendships. Davison & Neale (1982) suggest that 'of all the aspects of human suffering that command the attention of psychopathologists and clinicians, few touch the lives of more people than problems involving sex'. Many psycho-sexual disorders are perceived to stem from early learning and socialisation, treatment being offered ranging from aversion to social skills training.

An interest in social learning also leads to the study of personal and social perception. The cognitive structure within which a person thinks about himself, other people and events will determine the style and effectiveness of his behaviour. A structure which leads to feelings of helplessness or inadequacy may be a part of the picture presented by someone who is depressed (see Ch. 2). Therapists who have tried to apply these ideas within treatment refer to the need for cognitive restructuring. This involves suggesting to a patient alternative and positive ways of describing to himself what is happening or what events mean. For example, statements such as 'it does not matter if I fail as long as I know that I did my best', or 'I believe I am able to control the children's behaviour', can be rehearsed and invoked to help an individual to act in a more positive way when feeling stressed. Chapter 5 discusses these methods further.

The perspectives applied by a behaviourally oriented clinician to the problems of a client may be based on some or all of these ideas. Essentially he will be interested in the behaviour, its immediate antecedents and its consequences. This interest may extend to identifying current beliefs and attitudes which determine how someone will experience and respond to events.

The humanistic or existential view

Those who follow the lead given by Maslow and Rogers place stress on reality as it is experienced by the client. In order to share this reality a clinician must learn to empathise, or to adopt the other's phenomenological frame of reference. These terms are explained within Chapter 4 which is devoted to this topic because of its particular significance to occupational therapy.

Gestalt therapy, as described by Fritz Perls (Perls et al 1951), extends these ideas but differs slightly in its special emphasis on the present. Immediate experience and the comfortable satisfaction of current needs are made important; changes in behaviour are made by enhancing what an individual does and says and helping him to accept responsibility for these expressions.

Clinicians who are influenced by these ideas will be alert to the client's presentation of self, will be sensitive to freedom of will and expression, and will encourage self-determination. Solutions to problems are sought from within the client and not sought elsewhere in order to be prescribed.

The physiological view

Here we come full circle to the concept of disease, which was used earlier as an example of difficulties in descriptive terms. Terminology is important since the use, within psychiatry, of words associated with physical medicine influences the way in which we think about people and their problems. Maher (1966) demonstrates this very neatly by stating that: '[deviant] behaviour is termed *pathological* and is classified on the basis of *symptoms*, classification being called *diagnosis*. Processes designed to change behaviour are called *therapies* and are applied to patients in mental *hospitals*. If the deviant behaviour ceases, the patient is described as *cured*.'

Attempting to categorise people on the basis of their behaviour, their descriptions of how they think and feel and their personal history is difficult. The presence of any physical abnormality introduces a welcome degree of objectivity into the assessment which is being made. A physiological or medical approach describes distress as being the result of illness which, once identified, should be amenable to treatment. Strict adherence to this model assumes that conditions in which physiological abnormalities have not yet been discovered have been incompletely researched. Once the congenital abnormality, the virus, the traumatic damage or the chemical deficiency has been identified then the appropriate treatment can be developed.

It is very easy to criticise this 'medical' model of abnormal behaviour, indeed it is almost fashionable to do so. Here are examples of the types of ammunition which might be used:

When a disease model is applied to abnormal behaviour [however] it is often not possible to assess independently both the symptoms and the supposed cause of the symptoms. Certain behaviour or symptoms are categorised as mental illnesses and given names, but then the name of the illness itself is often cited as an explanation for or cause of these same symptoms. For example, a patient who is withdrawn and hallucinating is diagnosed as schizophrenic; however, when we ask why the patient is withdrawn and hallucinating, we are often told that it is because the patient is schizophrenic.

Davison & Neale 1982

Or, look at this suggestion, made in somewhat terser tone, by Coulter (1973):

Biogenic theorists of the aetiology of mental disorder cannot hope to achieve a statement of the necessary and sufficient conditions for the holding of some bizarre belief or the communication of some unusual experiences.

On the other hand, physiological psychiatry has an undeniable track record. Endocrine and metabolic disorders which used to lead to mental handicap are now recognised and treated. General paralysis of the insane has become a historic interest rather than a current problem. Genetic counselling is available to those who risk endangering their offspring with genetically transmitted forms of presenile dementia.

Examples of a second level of success can be seen in the control, by physical means, of psychological distress. Minor group tranquillisers, antidepressant and hallucinogenic drugs allow people to start to tackle problems again. Phenothiazine derivatives appear to make endurable the more bizarre aspects of psychosis or otherwise uncontrolled anxiety. Electroconvulsive treatment, more controversially, relieves states of depression in some people. These successes are rated as secondary for two main reasons. The first is that they ameliorate but do not cure and in some cases the reasons for their effectiveness are not fully understood. Secondly, they do not admit a possible 'chicken and egg' problem within psychiatry; do physiological abnormalities in the transmission of nerve impulses, which may be a feature of depressive illness, precede the disturbance of mood or are they a consequence of it? Are the abnormal levels of cortical arousal part of a pattern of malfunction which causes 'schizophrenic' behaviour or do they arise from some other more significant distress? The answers proposed to such questions are not quite convincing enough yet.

Another criticism of the medical model is that it is of more use to doctors and research workers than to patients and to other disciplines which seek to offer help. It gives rise to problems of diagnostic labelling without prescribing a clear course of ameliorative action. The worst tags are those such as 'personality disorder' which define abnormality in vague and abstract terms. The problem is retained in the province of medicine but physiological abnormalities are not sought with any vigour in the jungle of biographical disasters and personal failures.

Recapitulation

This chapter has so far failed to define mental illness but has posed some questions. It is hoped that these questions are more pertinent to a student of occupational therapy than a list of facts for easy memorisation would have been. This may sound like an excuse, but the most important thing that a professional education can give to you is an opportunity to join in the debate, to compare different viewpoints and to develop your own working philosophy. In order to do this, an occupational therapist must have a working knowledge of clinical psychiatry; a useful summary is not given here since many excellent textbooks are available. It is also essential to be able to apply knowledge about psychology to a function–dysfunction continuum and to integrate ideas from other disciplines, in particular sociology, into an understanding of what may be going on.

PRACTICAL PROBLEMS

Occupational therapists seek to assist people in practical ways. They are interested in the skills which an individual is able to draw upon when performing everyday tasks and also in the concepts and attitudes which affect his performance of roles. Occupational therapy is essentially a social process which is problem oriented. Its practitioners do not normally prescribe forms of activity or therapy on the basis of symptom or diagnosis.

There are a number of subjective experiences which are shared by a wide variety of clients and which contribute to their difficulties in both task and role performance. They tend, also, to be the experiences which are active in preventing the client from sharing perceptions of the social world with others, thereby excluding him from the personal contacts which arise out of a shared reality. Three important areas in which these experiences occur are disorders of perception, disorders of thought and disturbance of mood. It is difficult to think of any psychological disorder which does not involve at least one of these.

Disorders of perception

The process of perception involves organising and interpreting sensory stimuli. It is relatively straightforward if you think of it purely as a part of receiving information about the environment. Visual perception, for example, involves the translation of the retinal image of the object in my hand to the 'knowledge' that it is a black pen. Sensory inputs from other receptors are also translated and add to my current perception that the pen is light, warm and makes a noise as it travels across the paper. Using this level of description we can accept the definition of an hallucination as being a perception in the absence of any relevant external stimuli.

Thus, a visual hallucination involves 'seeing' something which is not physically present and an auditory hallucination hearing something although no sound is discernible by others. Hallucinations may involve any of the sensory modalities. Some people report 'combined' hallucinations where more than one sense is involved, but it would be unusual to report not only seeing a pink elephant but also smelling, tasting, touching and hearing it.

It is important to differentiate between hallucinations and illusions. The latter are a misinterpretation or 'misperception' of sensory information which is actually present. An everyday example would be a mirage, perceiving a pool of water on the road ahead when actually the visual information should have been interpreted as a combination of heat haze and the reflection of sun on tarmac. It is not the eye that is fooled but the brain, and psychologists spend hours producing pictures and models to demonstrate the extent to which we can be misled in our perceptions of perspective, distance, depth, colour and size.

The problem of describing perception, and then hallucination and illusion, as an extension of the sensory modalities is that this oversimplifies the process in a way which can be misleading in itself. Perception is an active process which includes the involvement of memory, expectations and mood, and attention as well as other factors not expanded upon here.

Recall

It is quite obvious that in order to identify a stimulus we compare it with information that has been 'stored' about previous experiences. This is not necessarily a conscious process. I can recognise my back door key amongst others on a ring but could not 'bring to mind' and describe its position on the ring, the shape of its indentations or the number engraved on it. I know it is a key, that is I can place it in a generalised family of differently shaped objects that are all called keys, and I know that it is my back door key because I can select its own particular features. What is more I can do it in the dark. All cognition must necessarily involve recognition. It is likely that the process is one of testing any novel pattern of stimuli against a series of hypotheses, actively searching for a reasonable interpretation.

Expectation and mood

We frequently see or hear that which we were expecting. This is one of the major reasons why we can be taken in by illusions. Geometrical illusions to be found in psychology textbooks often mislead us by using previous experiences of perspective or relative sizes and shapes in a context where they do not apply.

There is, however, another way in which expectations can affect perception. We can associate certain environments or situations with the likelihood of pleasant or unpleasant experiences. Walking down a dark street at night, with the knowledge of frightening things that have happened to others in just such a setting, how are you likely to perceive a sudden movement in the shadows or a light clicking noise? Escalating anxiety, and then panic, in such a situation can lead to seeing, hearing or feeling things which do not exist.

One's prevalent mood can also distort perception, or at least lead one's perceptions of the world to be out of tune with the perceptions of others. Scharfetter (1980) suggests that 'In depression, to a severely downcast and melancholy man his surroundings seem less lively, colourful, clear and distinct. Sometimes, it is as though he were experiencing them at a distance. A depressed patient may experience himself as falling to pieces; feeling putrefied, he may even smell the decayed odour that emanates from him'.

Attention

Accurate perception and the organisation of sensory input is reliant on some degree of selective attention to stimuli. To perceive every stimulus available to you simultaneously would be overwhelming and would result in not being able to give meaning to the environment at all. However, in order to select out certain stimuli which are to be perceived, it must be necessary to recognise all of them and to discard the irrelevant. This is illustrated by the well known 'cocktail party phenomenon', when you selectively attend to one conversation and are unaware of the content of others until your own name is mentioned. Whatever mechanism has been censoring out irrelevant stimuli has recognised a significant input and sent it up for attention. There has been considerable research in this field since Broadbent (1958) suggested the existence of an active filtering mechanism. Students of occupational therapy should pay particular attention to factors which may be responsible for the apparently anarchic experience of the world as perceived by those with 'psychotic conditions'. If a wide range of stimuli are competing for attention, and if we accept that some are selected and others determined to be irrelevant, then this raises important questions about the criteria used by any individual for the selection of relevant material. Both the interests and the mood of an individual will influence his selective attention to his environment. If you are expecting a guest, then you hear every car door that slams. If you are an ornithologist, you hear each new bird song. If you are in love, then you are aware of all stimuli that can be related, even tenuously, to your lover; and if you are feeling thoroughly 'got at', then every hostile nuance in the conversation of those around seems to be significant and personal. It is interesting to remember that last example when confronted by someone who is described as having paranoid ideas. Might it be that, in a social world which contains both hostility and tolerance, he is responding to events or comments which have not warranted your attention and you are perceiving the same world in a more positive and friendly way?

Summary

These comments on perception have been made because this is a particularly significant topic within psychiatry. Hallucinations are only one example of perceptual disorder. Equally important to the therapist are disturbances of body image, experiences of depersonalisation and derealisation and problems arising from faulty interpersonal perception. The topic of interpersonal perception, which includes the formation of impressions, the interpretation of mood and behaviour and the attitudes adopted by individuals within relationships, is a theme which runs through almost every chapter that follows. Cook (1979) sums up its significance: 'The way people see each other determines the way they behave towards each other, so the study of "person perception" is one of the keys to understanding social behaviour'.

Perception as a cognitive process and perception as a social influence have been referred to within this section. Unless you are a purist, in terms of psychological research into observable behaviour, it is permissible and useful to combine these perspectives in terms of mental illness. They are interlinked and complementary within any individual's attempt to make sense of his world.

Disturbance of thinking

It is not easy to separate thought and speech. One could say that thought is the process and speech the product through which thinking is expressed. However, it is difficult to rule out the possibility that the way people think is deeply influenced by their vocabulary and verbal ability. When people are unhappy or disturbed we realise their distress through the content of their speech and so, for simplicity, the two will be regarded here as a single dimension.

In order to think effectively an individual needs to know who he is, in what context he is operating and what he hopes to achieve. He needs to be able to refer to past learning and experiences to maintain concentration over a period of time and to interpret the environment and the responses of others. He needs to organise all of this information, to handle abstract as well as concrete concepts, to form hypotheses, to reason the possibilities and probabilities involved and to express this entire process in the signs and symbols which make up language. Cognition, or thinking, is therefore a very complex process which is reliant not only on intelligence but also on features which include perception, memory, attention, attitudes, concentration, creativity, reasoning and language. At every stage the process is vulnerable to disruption for a number of different reasons. Physical factors include altered consciousness, toxic states induced by metabolic disorder, deficiency, drugs or alcohol, and brain damage or deterioration. Emotional factors include debilitating anxiety, the blocking of information through the use of defence mechanisms, retardation due to depression, shock and fear. Social factors include immaturity, helplessness acquired through learning, features of socialisation, conflict, and other environmental influences. Whatever the reasons, disorders in thinking involve the following wide spectrum.

Consciousness

To be conscious is to know about oneself and about the world. This involves first of all being wakeful, secondly being lucid (that is able to relate clearly to the immediate environment) and thirdly being aware of oneself as a unique and enduring being against a background which includes reality, experience and time.

Wakefulness is essentially a function of the reticular formation, the hypothalamus and frontal lobes. Being essentially a state controlled by the mid-brain it can be affected by physical phenomena such as toxicity or brain damage. It is normally subject to fluctuations as each individual has patterns of sleeping and waking and of activity and non-activity. It is subject to the general state of an individual's physical health and can be disrupted by emotional experiences as different from one another as terror and boredom. Information about wakefulness can be gained not only from overt physical signs such as eye movements and muscle tone but also from electroencephalograms which measure the amount of cerebral electrical activity taking place.

Lucidity involves being able to make use of one's own perceptive, cognitive, intellectual and sensory function. The degree of lucidity is, of course, closely connected to the degree of wakefulness but involves understanding the environment as well as being aware of it. Information about lucidity is gained by questioning the patient about where he is, what he is doing and why he is doing it.

When problems related to consciousness occur, they are usually due to some temporary or permanent damage to the brain. Clouding of consciousness, drowsiness, confusion and delirium, for example, are all problems which are associated with organic conditions.

At the other end of the scale certain patients may describe states of heightened consciousness. Their understanding of the world seems to be intensely enriched and they report vivid sensory awareness and inspired thinking and feeling. Again, the reasons for these experiences are normally physiological, typically through taking stimulant or hallucinogenic drugs. A similar experience of general stimulation may be reported by patients who are described as suffering from 'mania' where the aetiology is less clear.

Memory

Memory is a complex process and is well documented within most basic psychology courses. Memory is the essential component of all perception, learning and reasoning. It also has a strong affective component which can be demonstrated by observing how motivation, stress or repugnance can influence forgetting.

An individual's biography, social identity, ability to deal with the present and capacity to have valid ambitions for the future are all invested in memory. Any damage to the ability to retain and recall information is therefore deeply threatening to a person and may give rise to secondary problems of denial, confabulation or emotional distress. Psychologists have distinguished between long- and short-term memory; both of these functions can be disturbed.

Organic factors leading to disturbance of memory can be recognised in the 'brain failure' of some elderly people and in those where the brain has been damaged by trauma or by toxic substances such as alcohol. The nature of the disturbance is related to the extent of the damage or deterioration but is often associated with the recall of recent information.

A sudden shock, such as a bang on the head, electroconvulsive treatment or an intense emotional experience may interfere with the processing and retention of recent information, leading to a memory gap. The period of time which is 'lost' in this way will vary with the severity of the shock.

Emotional elements in the maintenance of an effective memory are more difficult to explain. The phenomenon of total amnesia, which may be hysterical in origin, or may be a response to an unbearable degree of stress, is one extreme. Those patients who are depressed or anxious often complain of having a poor memory; they find difficulty in retaining both important and trivial details. Although it may be tempting to ascribe this problem to low levels of concentration and motivation, this does not really account for the degree of difficulty that such people are experiencing.

Thinking

This is an artificially broad heading since it could be taken as embracing all of cognition. The word is used here to mean the ability to examine information and to respond to it in an organised way. Thinking involves being able to use the symbols of language and speech coherently. To communicate our thinking to others we need to have symbols and a perception of reality in common with them. Disturbance of thinking can be recognised in a wide variety of disorders. Emotional disturbance can affect the speed of thought, depression of mood often leading to slowness and to difficulty in grasping new information. This should not be confused with a change in pace which is normal in old age and does not necessarily affect the quality of reasoning. In more acute conditions there may be difficulties in thinking clearly at all and the patient complains of blocks and breaks occurring in a train of thought, or he may get stuck in a loop of repetitive and unproductive ideas. Melancholy brooding as well as apparently psychotic perseveration may demonstrate this sort of problem.

A lack of control in thinking may also be described by patients or be observed form the content of their speech. A simple example of this is the 'flight of ideas' which arises from acceleration of thought to the extent that new material intervenes in the expression of every sequence, and superficial associations are formed. Other people complain that ideas are being imposed upon them from outside or are being withdrawn. This latter experience is very close to delusion.

Other disorders of thought involve degrees of apparent irrelevance or incoherence. It is difficult to assess how much of the difficulty lies in the processing of ideas and how much in expressive problems. What comes out may not sound either clear or logical but we can only guess from a person's speech, and from any indication of distress or frustration which accompanies this speech, the degree of disorganisation in the person's actual thinking.

Delusion

A delusion is a private, firmly held, and personally significant belief about the world. To this extent we may all claim to have a few. The textbooks tell us that a delusion becomes a psychiatric symptom when the beliefs encompassed within it are false. To say that something is false or untrue means that it is incompatible with reality as it is experienced and expressed by those of us who are not deluded. This is not a heretical attempt to obscure the issue, merely a warning that truth is relative. Those people who have disabling delusional beliefs find themselves isolated and alienated from the everyday experiences of other people. They may spend much time brooding over these ideas and may construe unrelated events as providing proof or evidence; in this way systems of delusional ideas are built up.

For some people the social world revolves around their own delusions. A central idea that they are extraordinary or historically significant persons colours all their relationships and perceptions. Others may be able to sustain delusional beliefs alongside an appreciation of the world as perceived by others, or may have isolated delusions which refer only to specific topics or situations. Delusions are not experienced only by those who are described as being psychotic; they are merely an extreme form of unshared belief which may arise from any form of emotional or physical isolation.

Disturbance of mood

It is easier for many of us to understand varieties in mood than to relate to disturbances in perception and cognition. Perhaps this is because we assume our own perceptions and thoughts to be similar to those of other people, whereas we know that our feelings fluctuate, are unpredictable to others and are, to ourselves, unique. We also know from experience that the running of many occupational therapy departments is subject to at least half a dozen uncoordinated menstrual cycles. It is acceptable, and sometimes comforting, to believe that one's mood is affected by physical facets such as physiological needs and the balance or imbalance of hormones. Any suggestion that our perceptions of the world and the way in which we think are subject to such arbitrary influences is curiously more threatening.

Patients who are experiencing difficulties associated with mood may be able to count on a greater degree of empathy from their therapists, but the relationship is still problematic. It is sometimes difficult to know what to say to someone whose misery or inappropriate reaction exceeds our own imagined response to a situation.

There are four major styles of affective disturbance which inhibit communication and relationship. These are:

- lability and rapid fluctuation in mood
- inappropriate emotional responses
- misery
- euphoria.

Lability and rapid fluctuation in mood. Emotional lability is typified by immediate reaction to every stimulus. The instantaneous way in which such reactions are produced make them appear superficial, and sometimes irrelevant. The mood invoked is often short-lived which leaves one, perhaps unfairly, questioning the validity of the emotions expressed. This style of emotional response is associated with immaturity, intellectual impairment and damage to the brain.

Inappropriate emotional responses. Inappropriate responses are those in which a topic or situation which would normally evoke one set of feelings gives rise to different and incompatible reactions. This is not an entirely abnormal phenomenon as any student, who has answered a classroom question wrongly and collapsed into a heap of giggling mirth, will know. The classic examples of inappropriate affect involve psychotic patients who receive bad news, for example of family bereavement, with apparent amusement. It is not uncommon, however, to find apparently normal people who cannot discuss traumatic periods within their own lives without smiling or laughing in an incongruous way. It is difficult to assess the extent to which such incongruity is the product of embarrassment or defensiveness, and to what extent the emotion felt is truly out of context with the circumstances. Just as thinking and language are difficult to separate, genuine feelings and expressed emotions may not complement each other. It is rarely effective to be impatient with those who find it difficult to represent their feelings accurately, nor is it relevant to determine what a person *should* feel within any set of circumstances. The decision as to whether to confront a person with his own inappropriate reaction, or to accept whatever emotional reaction he chooses to present, can only be made on an individual basis and in the light of knowledge about other treatment he may be receiving.

Misery. Misery is common enough as one of the main features of depressive illness. Extreme unhappiness and negative self-concept frequently occur in other disorders, even when they have not been identified as a major problem. Very few people who are in receipt of psychiatric treatment are consistently happy. Normal fluctuations in mood and fortune include periods of misery but, as sufferers, we retain the knowledge that most subjective experiences are short-lived. We know that things will get better, that we will not always feel so foul. Real misery is experienced when one loses touch with the fluid and cyclical nature of existence and comes to believe that there will be no unforeseeable change. It is a short step then to believing oneself undeserving of improved fortune and responsible for the surrounding waste and sadness. To be told to cheer up can contribute merely another ounce of guilt to the burden. It is difficult for a therapist, a nurse or a relative, to know how to cope with misery as expressed through tears and self-derogatory statements. We know enough to avoid denying them, which is to impede the formation of any relationship, or to reinforce them with the style of sympathy which encourages dependency and helplessness.

Euphoria. The patient who is euphoric or 'high' creates a variation on this problem for himself and for those around him. Extravagant behaviour may be exhilarating, embarrassing or dangerous. It is also exhausting for all concerned. Contrary to superficial descriptions, being high is not the opposite of feeling low. Both are expressions of isolation; both may have physiological antecedents or consequences. As with every other manifestation of psychological distress, the causes may be various but the outcome is social disruption.

REFERENCES

Arieti S, Bemporad J 1978 Severe and mild depression, the psychotherapeutic approach. Tavistock, London
Bandura A 1960 Relationship of family patterns to child behaviour disorders. Stanford University Press, Stanford
Cook M 1979 Perceiving others. Methuen, London
Coulter J 1973 Approaches to insanity. Martin Robertson, London
Davison C G, Neale J M 1982 Abnormal psychology, 3rd edn. John Wiley, New York
Maher B A 1966 Principles of psychopathology: an experimental approach. McGraw-Hill, New York
Perls F, Hefferline R F, Goodman P 1951 Gestalt therapy. Penguin Books, Harmondsworth
Scharfetter C 1980 General psychopathology. Cambridge University Press, Cambridge

2

Stress and vulnerability

Averil Stewart

INTRODUCTION

In the past, much research has linked illness to stress, as though there was a causal relationship (Lowe 1969, Dohrenwend & Dohrenwend 1974)—the greater the exposure to stress, the greater the likelihood of illness—but others (Gentry & Kobasa 1984, DeLongis et al 1988, Lydeard & Jones 1989) have recognised that this is not universal, nor is the impact constant. While individuals are all subjected to potential stress, some are more vulnerable than others, and more so at some times than others.

Each age in the development of man must have created stress and anxiety in relation to survival. For man, the hunter, catching the next buffalo depended on many things besides his own skill, and not least the winds and weather driving the herd in a specific direction. Survival depended on his success. The agrarian, industrial and now what might be called the technological revolution have all brought about changes to lifestyles with resulting winners and losers, successful copers and less fortunate people failing, through perhaps no direct fault of their own. A sense of failure, frustration at never seeming to win, constantly being presented with barriers, or threatened redundancy, or yet another directive for change, all may contrive to stress individuals to the point where mental health is in jeopardy or physical illness a sequel.

Why is it that experiences of stress and threats to our survival differ from person to person? Unfamiliarity of surroundings and fear may induce particularly high levels of stress for some patients admitted to hospital for the first time. Similarly, some students embarking on a new fieldwork placement may have higher levels of apprehension than others, perhaps depending on previous experiences as well as innate personality characteristics. Others appear less susceptible and more resilient.

This chapter will define stress, discussing positive and negative aspects, what causes it and how people often cope. Vulnerability and predisposing psychopathology will also be examined. Over the past two decades, there has been an increasing amount of research into risk and resistance, or protective factors and strategies for coping, hence this third edition has a considerably enlarged set of references worthy of following up. The ability to help people understand and cope with situations and their consequences, and to develop adaptive behaviours is inherent in occupational therapy. How people think and feel about themselves and the world in which they live are essential component of this process (Fine 1991).

WHAT IS STRESS?

Stress is a common experience but one that is hard to define in specific terms. Many other words such as 'anxiety' and 'tension' seem to be interchangeable. The word 'stress' originates from the physical sciences and means a 'constraining or impelling force' (Concise Oxford Dictionary), and 'effort' or a 'demand upon energy'. In this sense, stresses on structures have an optimum point when tension is maintained and breaking point is withheld. Too much stress and the wires will snap.

Tension in human terms can indicate power and strength as when muscles are tensed, ready for action. But it can also be a painful and subjective experience as when the brow is tense and a headache ensues. This suggests a feeling of discomfort and may be described as nervous tension, although long-term effects may be more serious leading, for example, to gastrointestinal problems or coronary heart disease.

In this chapter, stress is considered in its widest sense. As defined by Lazarus & Folkman (1984), it is the relationship between person and environment that is appraised by the person as taxing or exceeding his or her resources and endangering his or her well-being. The impact of stress is not a simple one-way process since individuals can be cushioned in different ways and to different degrees depending on a range of psychosocial factors and mechanisms. In other words, stress is a complex variable resulting from interdependent processes including susceptibility and resistance, and influenced by mediating factors such as cognitive appraisal and coping strategies which in turn affect the frequency, intensity and duration of psychological and somatic responses.

Stress as a positive force

Just as tension has an optimal level in mechanical terms so has stress. Many people thrive on stress and for some there is the potential to transform traumas into triumphs. At the optimal level for each individual it can be valuable. The literature on coping with stress gives evidence of how some people not only overcome adversity on their own but actually benefit from it (Taylor 1983, Fine 1991). For example, optimum personal levels of stress can keep us on our toes, spark off energy and the drive to achieve full potential. Without that specific and individual quota of stress some people function below par and can be slow and apathetic. How often are assignments left until the last minute for completion? For many, without that pressure which is brought by limited time, there is insufficient motivation to harness thoughts and organise words into acceptable scripts. As with the writer facing an empty page, so does the climber approaching a new pitch feel muscles tense ready for action and feel the senses alert, ready for all eventualities, while judgement is sharpened and decisions are made. Sometimes the monotony of everyday life causes individuals to test out those senses, in order to produce excitement and exhilaration and the feeling of power and achievement. Similarly, but at the other end of the scale, there are people with very demanding and potentially very stressful jobs who also seek out challenges in very different stress-provoking situations. These exciting, taxing activities, whether gambling, scrambling up mountains, or vandalising are generally within the control of the individual. Their successful outcomes provide individuals with, or reinforce, their own self-concept and ability to survive, as well as strengthening social relationships. The concepts of challenge and control in relation to surviving and coping with stress will be returned to later.

Stress-provoking situations

Stress is inevitable and for some may be a vital part of their experience with each new event provoking new challenges. For others, life's many and varied events bring their own stress and strain. Changing circumstances like one's first day at school bring exposure to new people, new systems of organisation, written and unwritten rules and the law of the playground. All this and more can be rather intimidating until one learns to cope and finds ways of ensuring survival. Taking examinations, the storms of adolescence, one's first job, leaving home, new roles and responsibilities, changing circumstances, emotional upheavals including illness and bereavement all take their toll, producing different levels of stress for each individual. These depend on the individual's threshold and how each perceives the world, as either threatening and destructive or supportive and caring. Stress can be cumulative as one trauma or tragedy is heaped on to other potentially stressful life events. Stress can be studied in relation to individuals and everyday life events, or the effects of major life events on populations affected by war, natural disasters or by imprisonment and torture. Experimental situations can also be created for the study of the effects of stress on animals or volunteers but despite rigorous control their applicability and explanatory value remains uncertain (Lydeard & Jones 1989).

Aetiology of stress

Many environments appear hostile to a happy and stress-free existence. Aetiology can be considered from a geographical, racial, historical perspective, or at a personal interpersonal level. At the high-risk environmental level, there are many examples of countries or local communities which are, or have been, war ridden, from South Africa and Ulster to Bosnia and Notting Hill Gate. Other circumstances include poverty, family instability and inadequate nutrition, and a combination of these can lead to unhealthy ways of coping. Resilience and protective defence mechanisms may include violence. While this may be one way of managing the stress, it in turn creates other stresses. Acts of violence, even when perceived as one's duty as part of war, create stress.

Studies of maternal stress and children's development (Rutter 1990), styles of parental rearing (Parker 1993), unemployment (McKenna & Payne 1989) and exposure to witnessing physical trauma (Classen et al 1993) yield further examples of high-risk environments which put individuals in potential danger.

Bereavement is a life event which affects us all and hence has been studied extensively. The saying 'to die of a broken heart' is not without its evidence. Parkes et al (1969) found that the mortality rate for widowers aged 55 and older during the first 6 months of bereavement was 40% higher than would have been expected for married men of the same age. The conclusion follows that an event such as losing one's wife leads to an increased mortality rate even if temporarily. The loss of an important person can be widened into the concept of 'deprivation of meaningful social contact' and include job loss, divorce and in general having fewer friends and social relationships. This concept does, however, raise questions about the nature of the relationships, their quality and endurance as well as quantity and significance, and about the characteristics of individuals which lead to meaningful or transient relationships.

When stressful situations are analysed, it would seem that a generalisation can be made in that acute stress occurs when there is a threat to one's identity or integrity, when there has been a change in status with a resulting change in role and before one's adaptive behaviour has been established. Temporarily, at least, the individual is not in control and lack of control leads to anxiety. If the stress is to be short-lived, the alerted senses will assist in dealing with the situation and control will be regained. However, if the stress is excessive and if no apparent changes in behaviour alleviate it, then energy and drive will be sapped and motivation to continue seeking alternative behaviours will be undermined and carry the potential for developing psychopathology.

While recognising different thresholds and causative factors, work has been done to establish stress scores, each weighted for perceived severity of the event.

Measuring stressful events

Early work by Holmes & Rahe (1967) involved identifying 43 events which could be considered as stress related. Interviews and questionnaires led to the assessment of the meaning of these events. Each event's potential for disruption and change was subsequently weighted, with remarkably high correlations for the ranked order of stressful events being obtained when tested across different cultural groups. However, later studies have suggested that simply counting the number of life events is as predictive of potential stress as are the more complicated weighted scores of the so-called life change units (Zimmerman 1983). While life event scales are useful as a means of indicating contextual stress, there are nevertheless a number of criticisms and potential for continued research into the multidimensionality of life event scales and the relations of these to outcomes (Pianta et al 1990).

There are many other studies, scales and inventories which consider general health and wellness issues in relation to stress. These contribute to the attempt to establish standardised measures of self-assessed health (Hunt et al 1986) and include the General Health Questionnaire (GHQ) with its insomnia, anxiety and depression subscales, Nottingham Health Profile (NHP) and the Hassles and Uplifts Scale, to name but three.

The NHP contains 38 statements covering six areas of perceived health: emotional reactions, pain, energy level, social isolation, physical mobility and sleep. The statements are presented in random order and the respondent is asked to indicate whether or not they apply at the present. Empirical weighting indicates their perceived severity with the overall score out of 100 indicating the level of dysfunction in the different domains (McKenna & Payne 1989).

A refined version of the Hassles and Uplifts Scale, used in an American study of 75 married couples in 1985, was part of a more comprehensive methodology which included other instruments to measure daily health, self-esteem and emotional support. The battery of questionnaires and monthly interviews over the 6-month period led to some not unsurprising findings, namely that there was a tendency for an increase in daily hassles to be associated with a decline in health and mood. Nevertheless, large individual variations in this relationship, with health and mood in some individuals actually improving when daily stress levels rose, were reported (DeLongis 1988). Furthermore, 'persons with low self-esteem and low emotional support had a higher probability of a positive association between stress and both physical symptoms and poor mood than did those who were high in these psychosocial aspects' (p. 492).

It can be seen from the above that there is no simple relationship between stress and responses to it. In one dimension there can be gradations of causative factors related to personal characteristics and the environment, yet the irony of it is that in the other dimension these very factors can lead, to a greater or lesser extent, to the ability to cope. In other words hassles one day can be uplifts the next.

Stress at the physiological level

Stress can escalate when one is tired, suffering from premenstrual tension, insomnia or from a specific illness. The immediate reaction of the sympathetic nervous system to stress is to prepare the body for 'fight or flight'. Blood pressure rises, the mouth dries, pupils dilate, there is sweating, irregular breathing, perhaps a lump in the throat, tightening of abdominal muscles and a generalised feeling of anxiety leading to action. Hormonal and chemical changes as a result of stress have had impact on prevention and treatment of stress, leading, for example, to relaxation techniques or medication.

Continual exposure, beyond individual thresholds, can have distressing physical concomitants, such as headaches, nausea, diarrhoea, raised blood pressure, coronary heart disease, myocardial infarction, or lead to complications in pregnancy, psychosomatic disorder, increased psychopathology including anxiety state, depression, alcoholism or even suicide.

The new discipline of psychoneuroimmunology is examining the impact of consciousness, moods and attitudes on the nervous system and the body's defences. Fine (1991) reports that living life at a mildly hectic pace and viewing it with a degree of optimism has a beneficial effect on one's immune system. There are different responses of the immune system in different individuals to different stress or emotional experiences. However, it is also possible through learned behaviour and the ability to anticipate unpleasant experiences, to reduce certain levels of anxiety or to resist the stress-provoking nature of specific situations. Successful coping helps to develop a positive self-concept, which can lead to future efforts that in turn produce mastery in difficult situations.

Psychological stress

Psychological stress, on an escalating scale, may range from boredom, irritation and dissatisfaction to loss of self-esteem, lack of control, anxiety, depression and neurosis, perhaps leading ultimately to suicide. Emotional responses to everyday hassles can influence relationships, which can lead to further deterioration or alienation, thereby setting up a vicious cycle. However, some people are more effective than others at regulating their distress. In other words, where symptoms are recognised, some individuals can either seek ways of changing the stressful situation or the way in which they handle it. It can therefore be argued that strategies for coping can lie within people themselves; but some appear more vulnerable than others.

WHAT IS VULNERABILITY?

Consultation of Roget's Thesaurus and the Concise Oxford Dictionary yields: susceptibility to injury, criticism; to be in danger, defenceless, at risk, exposed, forlorn, unsafe. The concept of vulnerability suggests a predisposition to disorder because such individuals have enhanced sensitivity to life stressors. There is, however, a continuum from susceptible individuals at one end, i.e. those who feel completely helpless, become passive and lose their ability to engage in any sort of activity which will aid their survival or restore self-esteem, to those who demonstrate resilience to potentially 'dangerous' situations at the other.

If vulnerability is to do with a predisposition to developing psychopathology, under what circumstances is this predisposition likely to arise and what is the evidence for it? What circumstances lead to individuals being in danger or defenceless and hence susceptible to stress? In physical terms, an invading bacterium is necessary for infection to develop, but its ability to infect will depend on the current state of resistance or vulnerability of its potential host. A number of variables can moderate the effects and hence obscure the relationship between life events and physical disorder.

The classic study by Brown & Harris in 1978, on the social origins of depression, found that women experiencing the following were more likely to develop depressive symptoms:

- early loss of mother
- having three children or more
- lack of employment
- lack of a confiding relationship.

Subsequent development of this view indicates that the events in isolation are not responsible for the disorder but only in association with continuing difficulties and accumulating life stressors, or provoking events. In other words, these external factors exert influence on other psychological aspects such as self-esteem, which in turn affects adaptive behaviours.

The more recent research of Rodgers (1991) followed up individuals born in March 1946, who were identified from the Medical Research Council's National Survey of Health and Development (NSHD). The nature of Rodgers' survey made it possible to compare information with much of that obtained by Brown & Harris. Interestingly, loss of mother and having three or more children did not appear to be factors contributing to vulnerability. This may be as a result of changes to social mores and attitudes to single-parent families. However, financial hardship had a much more striking relationship with symptomatology and particularly when combined with a high-risk index derived from childhood (Rodgers 1991). In a similar way, anomalous parenting experiences in childhood have been shown to lead to low self-esteem and a related dysfunctional style of behaviour, but the links with a predisposition to depression are less strong (Parker 1993).

A number of models, as above, suggest that depression can be the expression of a combination of exogenous factors accompanied by psychological characteristics resulting from stressful events in vulnerable people. There is, however, another model that suggests that vulnerability can lead to disorder in the absence of a provoking agent, i.e. that even in those for whom life is not particularly stressful, trivial events can be exaggerated, producing overreaction or prolongation and frequent recurrence, thereby leading to morbidity and a chronic disorder. There is no simple explanation for interrelationships between external and internal factors, yet some people, despite being subjected to high levels of risk, are remarkably resilient.

WHAT IS RESILIENCE?

Resilience can be seen as the opposite of susceptibility. It is the positive aspect of adaptation in people at risk due to cumulative environmental stressors, but it need not be a fixed attribute. Individual and family differences play critical roles in personal achievements and mastery of the environment despite stressful events. Families can create very positive and supportive networks despite enormous external disadvantage, and parent–child relationships become key factors in adjustment to potential stressors.

Supportive families can be described as protective mechanisms, helping to reduce the threats and avoid what might become a maladaptive response. In a similar way, planning, discussion and controlled exposure to stressful situations which fall within a child's ability and understanding can help to develop coping mechanisms for the future. The alternative is overprotection and sheltering the child with the possibility of merely delaying an adverse reaction.

Resilience, or adaptive functioning, therefore stems from personal characteristics, previous experience, developmental history and the family and social context within which the child is brought up. Resilience, protective factors and the development of competence in the face of adversity have become important areas in the field of psychiatric risk research (Rutter 1990). These ideas are of considerable relevance to occupational therapists and long argued for by Adolf Meyer whose 'psychobiological approach placed emphasis on the importance of person–environment interactions at these key turning points in people's lives' (quoted in Rutter 1990, p. 182).

HOW DO PEOPLE COPE?

This section will look at mechanisms for coping with stress and reducing the impact of risk factors. Coping is primarily a psychological concept reflecting the personal balancing of internal resources and distressing emotions with external demands, potential risks and conflicts.

The appraisal model of coping

The person who becomes aware of stress building up, and recognises tension in muscles, may seek to avoid the situation and withdraw, or to adopt behaviour which will enable continuance. Some will seek temporary escape in a trip to the pub or a holiday further afield, while others will work off tension through sport or perhaps digging the garden. Deep breathing exercises and relaxing with a nice cup of tea can also help restore the body's equilibrium through physical intervention.

The appraisal model of coping depends first on cognitive appraisal, which is the process of interpretation that gives events specific meaning to each individual. Primary appraisal, as initially discussed by Lazarus & Folkman in 1984 and 1987 (quoted in Gage 1992), is the determination of the nature of what is happening in relation to inherent dangers or otherwise for the individual. Secondary appraisal concerns the individual evaluating his or her ability, strategies and resources as being sufficient to enable successful handling of the situation and averting the threat. Many factors interrelate to influence the impact of the primary cognitive/perceptual stage on the secondary evaluative/problem solving stage, thereby leading to the development of a coping plan with outcome and subsequent feedback mechanisms conveying success or failure (Gage 1992). Coping is a process which may or may not lead to mastery, since some situations indeed have to be tolerated and endured, but it does involve effort on the part of the individual.

Reduction of the impact of risk

While all are faced with risks in varying form, their impact can be lessened by anticipation and careful planning, for example by preparing a child for admission to hospital through other, happier separation experiences within a more secure environment. Educational input prior to major turning points in one's life, whether associated with the birth of the first child, or with retirement, can alleviate potential stresses.

Similarly to face the subject of death and separation from a loved one, rather than treating death as a taboo subject, can help the key players come to terms with the event and imagine ways of coping despite the loss. Cultural and religious beliefs as well as the phenomenon of hope can be critical mediating variables in the successful adjustment to stressful events, personal and social resources and to health. The study of Farran & McCann (1989), while limited to a small sample, gives evidence to suggest that maintaining hope in older people who are already hopeful, and identifying means of regaining it in those who have lost the sense of hope, can influence mental health.

Unconscious mechanisms for dealing with stress

Besides conscious strategies as described above, the subconscious mind also makes use of what Freud called 'defence mechanisms'. These are attempts by the ego to reduce anxiety and threats to the individual's self-esteem. Their use seems to be universal and for many they enable a state of health to be maintained. For others, however, the reduction of tension may not resolve the problem and indeed, according to psychoanalytic theory, can be considered as immature responses with potential to lead to psychopathology and eventual neurotic breakdown. There appears to be a lack of objective evidence in support of this claim, but nevertheless an understanding of the concepts does help in understanding the behaviours of some patients.

The number of defence mechanisms and their differentiation is controversial but the following descriptions of repression, denial, rationalisation, projection and sublimation serve as examples.

Repression. Memories and facts which are painful for the individual may be removed from conscious awareness and become repressed, thereby protecting the individual. However, there is some confusion between the use of the words 'repression' and 'suppression' and some debate ongoing as to which refers to actively pushing an unpleasant thought aside, such as forgetting an impending and potentially painful dental appointment, and which is more to do with inner feelings and conflicts. On the whole it appears that the historical use of repression for the unconscious process is the word which prevails.

Denial. Readers can also be excused for thinking that denial is similar to repression. However, denial is used to refer to distortion of the facts, and to a failure to believe and accept information which has been given; hence, in the individual's perception, it removes the problem. Denial of a diagnosis of cancer, for example, could be positive in terms of attempting to continue to live life normally; alternatively it can be seen as a strategy with limited chance of success, for it only postpones acknowledgement of the reality.

Rationalisation. Rationalisation takes place when the blame for failure is shifted on to something else. 'A poor workman blames his tools.' 'There are not enough staff to treat everyone properly.' These are not necessarily true or rational excuses but they make us feel better and help to justify conduct so that behaviour is excused. Rationalisation acts as a buffer from criticism but also prevents individuals from facing reality.

Projection. Projection, as the word suggests, means attributing to another, weakness within oneself. Rather than expose and admit to undesirable traits, they are ascribed to others. Hence, a mean person may claim that his or her meanness is solely in response to others; or 'everyone is so unfriendly, I am always on my own' may refer to the fact that it is the individual who initially conveys a hostile attitude towards others.

Sublimation. Sublimation is perhaps one of the most successful defence mechanisms, for it channels unacceptable motives into socially acceptable behaviour. Aggressive outlets may be found in sporting activities; a subconscious desire to have a child may direct this instinctive energy into caring for others and so remove possible frustration and tension.

Other defence mechanisms include reaction formation and displacement.

Personality characteristics

The development of personality has long fascinated philosophers, psychologists and others. Many different classifications have been described, but it is easier to describe different types than to account for the differences. The teachings of Hippocrates and Galen linked body chemistry to emotion. This makes sense in relation to excessive anxiety causing ulcers, loss of weight and increased activity of bowel and bladder. Hippocrates (5 AD) taught that the body was composed of four elements: air, water, fire and earth. Galen (2 AD) said that these elements corresponded to substances in the body: blood, phlegm, yellow and black bile; and, depending on the quantity of each within each individual, so did the personality differ. Four categories were identified, namely sanguine, phlegmatic, choleric and melancholic. However, since there are many different characteristics by which individual personalities can be judged, and since moods vary according to context of circumstances, it is extremely difficult to group people objectively into four types. Yet to have a framework of personality types does lead the therapist towards a better understanding of the individual. Jung and Eysenck have added the dimensions of introversion–extroversion and stable–unstable respectively. The continua, in two different directions as offered by these theorists, give a much greater range of traits and scope for categorisation. If, in fact, both ancient and modern theories are combined, a schematic diagram allowing for greater variation and understanding is produced (Fig. 2.1).

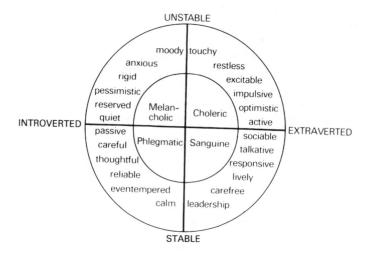

Figure 2.1 Modified from Eysenck & Rachman (1970).

Type A and Type B personalities

More recent studies of personality introduce the Type A and Type B personalities. Behaviour of the former tends to be competitive with intense commitment to vocational goals, restless, pressed for time, impatient and ambitious, whereas the latter is more passive and relaxed. Type A behaviour, not surprisingly, has been linked to high stress levels and the risk of cardiovascular problems is almost twice that for those categorised as Type B. However, since a large proportion of Type A do not develop excessive levels of stress despite their personality traits, a number of questions arise as to what the difference might be. Recent studies by Heilbrun & Friedberg (1988) have raised questions about mediating and predisposing factors. These relate:

- to self-preoccupation as a contributor to stress vulnerability by reducing self-esteem
- to repression as a defence strategy which becomes maladaptive
- to the level of self-control which can protect individuals
- to whether or not there are gender differences between highly stressed Type As and those thriving on the stress-evoking situations.

Although Heilbrun & Friedberg's research (1988) has focused on ambitions in American higher education students the findings are nevertheless of interest, namely that 'Type A behaviour, at least the hard-driven competitive, time-urgent variety that has been linked to stress and CHD [coronary heart disease] risk, seems to manifest itself in men who show deficiencies in self-control and in women whose self-control is superior' (p. 430).

Hardiness

The aspect of control has also been researched by Kobasa and co-workers in relation to the concept of hardiness as a personality style which appears to mediate against stress. The three key components of hardiness are:

- a sense of personal control over events and a belief in one's own ability to influence causes and solutions
- a strong sense of commitment to whatever one is doing
- an ability to see situations in positive terms of representing exciting challenges (Gentry & Kobasa 1984).

Such people appear to enjoy change and have learnt how to cope with the unexpected. Research carried out on a population of highly stressed business executives showed that high-stress/low-illness executives were hardier than high-stress/high-illness counterparts. Earlier research by Kobasa in 1982 (Gentry & Kobasa 1984) revealed other mediating factors in the life of stressed out business men, namely the benefit of regular physical exercise.

Measuring personality

There are many different personality inventories and factor analyses. They have often been criticised as being unreliable but there is increasing evidence of their usefulness. For example, results from over 15 000 adolescents between 1948 and 1954 on the Minnesota multiphasic personality inventory (MMPI) were followed up in 1987 in relation to subsequent development of schizophrenia. Findings suggested that those with early onset of schizophrenia could have been predicted from their substantially more disturbed ratings on the MMPI-associated characteristics of depression, withdrawal, anxiety, internal anger and social alienation, compared with those who developed schizophrenia much later in life and with normative controls (Hanson et al 1990). The depression scale in the MMPI will also help to identify not only those individuals who are sick enough to need psychiatric attention but also those whose depression is hidden from casual observation and is masked or called 'smiling depression'.

Learned behaviour as a means to coping

It has already been suggested that developing a form of self-control can influence levels of stress. Facilitating such development becomes an important role for therapists and was evident during the Persian Gulf War when combat stress led to the utilisation of occupational therapy and clarified its contribution for future wartime missions. In this situation army occupational therapists provided opportunities, based on the army's broader behavioural science approach, for individuals to learn to control combat stress, with purposeful activity being a principal factor in coping with stress (Ellsworth et al 1993).

Involvement in purposeful activity helps to maintain or restore self-esteem and hence can be an important coping strategy. Nelson Mandela describes how he managed to cope with the stresses of imprisonment and no doubt avoid the dangers of succumbing to passivity or, worse still, depression. He adopted a strategy which enabled him to take satisfaction in mundane activities, such as organising his cell on Robben Island to conserve as much space as possible. 'The same pride one takes in more consequential tasks outside prison one can find in doing small things inside prison.' (Mandela 1994, p. 475). In other words he took control, maintained a commitment to achieving goals no matter how small and saw a challenge in each task.

Just as coping can be learnt and have impact under certain conditions, so can the opposite be reinforced. If people are unable to escape from frightening, painful or stressful situations despite much effort, they may become helpless and passive, and such a negative concept of personal powerlessness can infiltrate other behaviours. Thus individuals begin to fail to discriminate between those circumstances in which they are truly helpless and those where they can take control. The intention of current legislation and the empowerment of individuals is intended to give a sense of purpose and responsibility for making decisions. The reality as opposed to the rhetoric remains to be seen. Will individuals have choice? Is society tolerant enough to let people live in a variety of non-conforming ways? The following description of an ex-alcoholic patient highlights the boundaries between helplessness and home-lessness. For Nick, sleeping under an upturned boat and working hard to survive each day was more of a challenge than the apparently more comfortable state which should have followed being given a place in a hostel. A roof over his head and regular meals in fact took away from his personal identity. He was expected to conform. He lost control of what he wanted to do and in the absence of other meaningful employment resorted back to the bottle.

PSYCHOPATHOLOGICAL EFFECTS OF STRESS

Already many references have been made to people who are not in control of their circumstances, who are less self-disciplined and less comfortable with themselves and others, who are unable to externalise feelings to produce anger or laughter and who lack environmental support. The potential relationship between causative factors, psychological problems and their expression is complex but may lead to one of a number of diagnoses: anxiety state, obsessive–compulsive disorder, conversion reaction, depression, phobia, dissociation, addiction or perhaps suicide, to name a few. Whatever neurotic label is given, behaviour in general leads to withdrawal from threatening, stressful circumstances into a more predictable world, whether through resorting to irrational fears of illness or through the apathy of depression. The neurotic person is often preoccupied with old events and people. The symptomatology and diagnosis will depend to a large extent on the susceptibility of the personality, the nature of the life event and other predisposing features with the severity being mediated according to more positive variables.

Details of the above diagnostic categories can be found in many psychiatric texts. More recent information and relevant findings arise from a paper by Classen et al (1993) which focuses on trauma and dissociation. Trauma, whether war or rape, road traffic accident or natural disaster, produces an abrupt physical change with loss of control and invariably subsequent symptoms of depression and anxiety. Trauma victims can develop a state of absolute help-lessness as a result of the world suddenly becoming unpredictable and threatening. The loss of personal control, whether physical, emotional or cognitive, makes it difficult for the individual to make sense of the experience and hence a state of consciousness known as dissociation develops.

Dissociative disorders

These disorders result in a disturbance or alteration in the normally integrative functions of identity, memory and consciousness and may take different forms. Each response, depending on the severity and duration of the initial trauma, is a way of distancing oneself from the event and may lead to feelings of depersonalisation or realisation. Amnesia is perhaps the most extreme dissociation state and a form of repression which has been so successful in cutting out the painful memories that it also removes awareness of personal identity. Anxiety symptoms are more common and less severe but nonetheless disabling in terms of difficulty in concentrating, insomnia, jumpiness and physical symptoms such as tachycardia or fatigue.

Acute stress disorder

This is a new diagnostic category proposed for the American Psychiatric Association DSM-IV, as reported by Classen et al (1993), and covers symptoms which continue to interfere with social or occupational functioning after the trauma and for as long as 1 month. During this period, counselling becomes important in order to help the people concerned to develop insight which will help reduce the psychological pain, remove any self-blame and help integrate the experience into something which can become tolerated. There is a major difference here in terms of therapeutic intervention compared with helping people to adapt to other stressful events and the subsequent symptomatology. In the former, the trauma survivor needs help to reduce potential for self-blame, whereas, in the latter, the individuals need to be helped to assume more responsibility. In both situations there is an important role for developing supportive relationships. Social networks can be one of the most powerful therapeutic tools in helping individuals to cope with stress. The question arises, however, of how one can reach those who are the least sociable or who are unlikely to stretch out towards that potential support.

Suicide and attempted suicide

Suicide is hardly a symptom but a pretty drastic piece of overt behaviour intent on destroying the self and so escaping from stress into oblivion without caring about the outcome. If on the other hand self-poisoning or self-injury is unsuccessful and in fact was never truly serious, then it is often seen as a 'cry for help' and perhaps as an attempt to manipulate people who are significant to the individual. Suicide is more common amongst those who are single, childless, alcoholic, isolated, unemployed, for whom hope for the future has been lost and who lack religious beliefs. The classic study by Durkheim, *Le Suicide*, published in France in 1897, identified suicide as being higher amongst Protestants than Catholics, higher for soldiers than civilians, higher in times of peace, prosperity and recession than during war and revolution or periods of economic stability. In other words, the social context within which suicide is committed leads to an understanding of the causation, although there are many different reasons for committing suicide. While socio-cultural factors have an important role to play, Durkheim suggested a fundamental factor was the degree of social integration into group life and the number of social ties which determined whether or not the person would be motivated to commit suicide. The corollary is that the level of social support and network of contacts that individuals have can help sustain them through periods sufficiently distressing to promote such a self-destructive act.

CONCLUSION

In this chapter, much has been written about stress and vulner-ability, the susceptibility and resilience of individuals and how mediating factors and coping strategies can buffer the individual against the possibility of developing psychopathology. More could have been written about the actual psychopathology but the serious reader is encouraged to seek more detailed evidence from such sources as Gentry's *Handbook of Behavioural Medicine* (1984) and Rolf et al's edited text on *Risk and Protective Factors in the Development of Psychopathology* (1990), along with numerous journal articles. Suffice it to add here that the role for occupational therapy is very clear, given the profession's emphasis on enabling people to develop adaptive behaviour and to enhance self-esteem and social competencies. Given our knowledge of risk factors, it should be possible to contribute to preventive strategies and so avoid later development of dysfunctional behaviour. With the expansion of community care and closure of psychiatric hospitals it becomes even more important to identify those more vulnerable within society. As Grossman (1991) says, albeit in relation to America, 'prevention programs should be offered in community organizations such as day-care centres, schools, neighbourhood centres, the workplace, senior citizen centres and private practice locations. Occupational Therapists are beginning to work in these settings and to engage in population-based planning but these remain isolated initiatives' (p. 39).

Action research to evaluate such initiatives will be essential, as too will the continuation of investigations into the links between psychopathology and life-span development, in order that models can be generated which will contribute predictive validity. In addition, Garmezy (1990) recommends that the construct of 'coping' needs to be explored in order to produce instruments for its measure and hence the standardisation of data which would enable valid and reliable study of an individual's reaction to truly stressful conditions. Such a step would move knowledge forward beyond many of the generalisations which have been written as though they were the truth. The whole subject is complex and statements must be treated with caution.

REFERENCES

Brown G W, Harris T O 1978 Social origins of depression: a study of psychiatric disorder in women. Tavistock, London
Classen C, Koopman C, Spiegal D 1993 Trauma and dissociation. Bulletin of the Menninger Clinic 57(2): 179–194
Courtney C, Escobedo B 1990 A stress management program, in patient-to-out-patient continuity. American Journal of Occupational Therapy 44(4): 306–310
DeLongis A, Folkman S, Lazarus R S 1988 The impact of daily stress on health and mood, psychological and social resources as mediators. Journal of Personality and Social Psychology 54(3): 486–495
Dohrenwend B S, Dohrenwend B P (eds) 1974 Stressful life events, their nature and effects. Wiley, New York
Ellsworth P D, Sinnott M W 1993 Utilisation of occupational therapy in combat stress control during the Persian Gulf war. Military Medicine 158: 381–385
Eysenck H J, Rachman S 1970 Dimensions of personality. In: Semenoff B (ed) Personality assessment. Penguin, Harmondsworth
Farran C J, McCann J 1989 Longitudinal analysis of hope in community-based older adults. Archives of Psychiatric Nursing 3(5): 272–276

Fine S B 1991 Resilience and human adaptability, who rises above adversity? 1990 Eleanor Clarke Slagle Lecture. American Journal of Occupational Therapy 45(6): 493–503

Gage M 1992 The appraisal model of coping, an assessment and intervention model for occupational therapy. American Journal of Occupational Therapy 46(4): 353–362

Garmezy N 1990 Reflections on the future. In: Rolf J et al (eds) Risk and protective factors in the development of psychopathology. Cambridge University Press, New York

Gentry W D, Kobasa S C O 1984 Social and psychological resources mediating stress–illness relationships in humans. In: Gentry W D (ed) Handbook of behavioural medicine. Guildford Press, New York

Grossman J 1991 A prevention model for occupational therapy. American Journal of Occupational Therapy 45(1): 33–41

Hanson D R, Gottesman I R, Heston L L 1990 Long-range schizophrenia forecasting: many a slip twixt cup and lip. In: Rolf J et al (eds) Risk and protective factors in the development of psychopathology. Cambridge University Press, New York

Heilbrun A F, Friedberg E B 1988 Type A personality, self-control, and vulnerability to stress. Journal of Personality Assessment 52(3): 420–433

Holmes T H, Rahe R H 1967 The social readjustment rating scale. Journal of Psychosomatic Research 2: 213–218

Hunt S M, McEwen J, McKenna S P 1986 Measuring health status. Croom Helm, London

Larson K B 1990 Activity patterns and life changes in people with depression. American Journal of Occupational Therapy 44(10): 902–906

Lazarus R S, Folkman S 1984 Coping and adaptation. In: Gentry D W (ed) Handbook of behavioural medicine. Guildford Press, New York

Lowe G R 1969 Personal relationships in psychological disorders. Penguin, Harmondsworth

Lydeard S, Jones R 1989 Life events, vulnerability and illness, a selected review. Family Practice 6(4): 307–315

McKenna S P, Payne R L 1989 Comparison of the General Health Questionnaire and the Nottingham Health Profile in a study of unemployed and re-employed men. Family Practice 6(1): 3–8

Mandela N 1994 Long walk to freedom. Little Brown, London

Parker G 1993 Parental rearing styles, examining the links for personality vulnerability factors for depression. Social Psychiatry and Psychiatric Epidemiology 28: 97–100

Parkes C M, Benjamin B, Fitzgerald R G 1969 Broken heart, a statistical study of increased mortality among widowers. British Medical Journal 1: 740–743

Pianta R C, Egeland B, Sroufe L A 1990 Maternal stress and children's development: prediction of school outcomes and identification of protective factors. In: Rolf J et al (eds) Risk and protective factors in the development of psychopathology. Cambridge University Press, New York

Rodgers B 1991 Models of stress, vulnerability and affective disorder. Journal of Affective Disorders 21: 1–13

Rolf J et al (eds) 1990 Risk and protective factors in the development of psychopathology. Cambridge University Press, New York

Rutter M 1990 Psychosocial resilience and protective mechanisms. In Rolf J et al (eds) Risk and protective factors in the development of psychopathology. Cambridge University Press, New York

Taylor S E 1983 Adjustment to threatening events, a theory of cognitive adaptation. American Journal of Psychology 41: 1161–1173

Taylor S E 1984 Issues in the study of coping, a commentary. Cancer 53: 2312–2315

Zimmerman M 1983 Weighted versus unweighted life event scores. Is there a difference? Journal of Human Stress 30: 30–35

FURTHER READING

Gentry W D (ed) 1984 Handbook of behavioural medicine. Guildford Press, New York
Keable D 1989 The management of anxiety. Churchill Livingstone, Edinburgh
Kendell R E, Zealley A K (eds) 1983 Companion to psychiatric studies, 3rd edn. Churchill Livingstone, Edinburgh
Madders J 1985 Stress and relaxation, 3rd edn. Martin Dunitz, London
Totman R 1979 Social causes of illness. Souvenir Press, London

3

The elderly client

Gillian Aspinall

INTRODUCTION

Since the publication of *The Rising Tide* by the Health Advisory
Service in 1982 there has been considerable development of
specialist services to elderly people with mental health problems
in Britain. In many areas they represent the most advanced
models of community psychiatry and are well placed to take good
advantage of the recent health service and community care
reforms. Recognising the need to harness the full skills of the multidisciplinary team, most of these new services include occupational therapy within them. Building on the work of therapists
who had worked in often isolated positions, occupational therapists
have developed their knowledge in establishing a model of work
in this interesting and challenging speciality of psychiatry.

This chapter presents a series of issues relevant to occupational
therapists working in the field of old age psychiatry today.

CONTEXTS OF SERVICE

Specialism versus ageism

Does the setting up of discrete services for people on the basis of
their age constitute the creation of a speciality or does it separate

elderly people from mainstream services? Could such a policy even be ageist? The attribution of the same characteristics, status and needs to a heterogeneous group that has been artificially homogenised, packaged, labelled and marketed as 'the elderly' shows that even well-intentioned policy may be framed by a subtle ageism (Neugarten 1970).

Ageist attitudes are institutionalised in our society. Cultural stereotypes in literature and television focus on loss and declining abilities, such as memory, physical attractiveness, speed and sexual prowess. These images tell us what it is to be old. Professionals and policy makers are not immune from this process and will have constructed their own view of old age from the myths, language and images presented to them throughout their personal and professional lives. An elderly person's own ageist attitude may prevent him or her seeking help from health services when it is needed, believing that even serious and preventable illnesses are merely due to age. Many elderly people are active and creative managers of their illness for some time before presenting for treatment.

The political background to the setting up of specialist services for mental health in old age is one of high unemployment and growing numbers of elderly people. These demographic changes are presented as a vast population of helpless elderly people who will require looking after by younger, more productive members of society. The move towards the introduction of market forces into the National Health Service has made elderly people 'customers'. Given that they represent a considerable proportion of the NHS's workload, this should in theory have placed them in a more powerful position. In reality, market forces seem to be influenced by more pragmatic considerations such as accessibility of services.

The development of specialist services recognises that expert assessment, diagnosis and treatment of the mental health problems presenting in old age is vital. An example of this is disorientation, a feature of dementia, which may also be due to vitamin B_{12} deficiency, toxic confusional states and depression. Other factors which characterise old age psychiatry are:

- an early epidemiological perspective
- emphasis on domiciliary assessment and treatment
- a commitment to continuing care
- the forging of links with other community agencies.

Undertaking initial assessments in the client's own home environment is in contrast to other medical specialities where initial contact is more often in a clinic. Community-based assessment, whilst more challenging in time and cost, ensures that difficulties are identified within their context and that carers and family members are involved from the outset. Similarly, links with other statutory and voluntary agencies are important if intervention is to be community focused and give continuity of care for clients. One of the aims of the National Health Service and Community Care Act 1990 was to ensure that 'the boundaries between primary health care, secondary health care and social care do not form barriers as seen from the perspective of the user'.

Community mental health teams

Arie (1985) described the multidisciplinary team as the linchpin of services to old age psychiatry. With an emphasis on outward-looking or community-based services many areas have established mental health teams for the elderly. To be effective and available to clients and carers, the team needs to employ flexible working patterns and ensure good communication and critical thinking between all professional groups. The team is typically made up of a consultant in old age psychiatry, community psychiatric nurse, clinical psychologist, social worker, physiotherapist and occupational therapist. There are a number of models of practice for community teams which reflect the varying levels of contact and cooperation between team members. For example:

- Referrals are received by the consultant and, after this medical assessment, are passed on to an appropriate member of the team. Reviews are held with that team member and the consultant. The team is merely a number of individuals with responsibility within a given geographical area.

- Referrals are discussed by all team members where it is decided which one is the most appropriate person to undertake the initial assessment. This is then presented at the next team meeting and a treatment plan agreed. Training is required to enable all team members to undertake initial assessments and flexible hours are needed in order to respond to urgent referrals.

The role of the occupational therapist

Core skills specific to the occupational therapist should be outlined and other skills which may lead to shared roles within the
team agreed. Lines of responsibility and management should
also be clear from the outset. Referring agencies, such as general
practitioners, will need information on the specific roles of group
members in order to refer appropriately to the team. For example,
a GP anticipating difficulties in the home will be able to refer the
patient to the occupational therapist for preventive work before a
crisis occurs.

A major focus of community occupational therapy is to help
the client restructure occupational activities and to adapt the
environment to allow for maximum independence. In the home
setting family members and others are intimately involved in the
treatment process. Ongoing family dynamics are affected by the
client's illness and must be considered in the therapy process.
Where a client is unable to adapt his or her behaviour in order to
increase independence, the main emphasis will be on the restructuring of the environment.

The assessment process should focus on the strengths and
difficulties of the client and carer in the context of their particular
environment and taking into account their goals and values. If,
for example, the goal is to remain in his or her home following a
bereavement, then, with the client, the occupational therapist
will need to identify areas of difficulty and design a treatment
programme to deal with them.

The assessment of independence in activities of daily living
should include all relevant activities for the client, the interaction
between physical, psychological and social factors and the
impact of these on the client's independence. For example, a
client suffering from depression may have significant difficulties
in preparing a meal, due to a sense of hopelessness and difficulty
in concentration. The approach, therefore, will need to focus on
the mental health difficulties underlying a particular behaviour,
but at the same time taking note of any associated physical
problems.

Another important area to be included in the assessment process
is that of socialisation. A supportive network of friends and
social contact is an important factor in maintaining life in the
community. Conversely, isolation and loneliness play a significant
role in difficulties encountered in coping with mental health

problems. The occupational therapist will need to suggest strategies to increase opportunities for socialisation.

The acute assessment ward

For some clients, admission to an acute ward will be necessary in order to assess the person's mental health problem or in order to commence treatment. In most areas separate wards exist for functionally ill clients and those with organic conditions, due to the differing environments and treatment regimes appropriate to each client group. Depression and dementia may co-exist and therefore accurate assessment as an inpatient may only be possible in some cases. Occupational therapists are members of the ward team and contribute to the assessment and treatment process.

Clients are seen for individual sessions in order to assess strengths and problems, devise a treatment programme and work on identified areas. Group sessions are also undertaken, with the client's programme directing him or her to specific groups.

Emphasis is on regaining ability and the re-establishment of roles and routines or on the introduction of new strategies and roles. Occupational therapy will be focused on the client's own home environment so that new skills and outlooks can be transferred on discharge. Home visits are undertaken in order to assess the client's ability to cope at home. Programmes of graded discharge and follow-up are important in preventing problems of adjustment to discharge from hospital, or readmission.

Day hospitals

With the emphasis on treatment and support for client's in the community many people are seen in day hospitals. In addition to the assessment of mental health problems, Cirirelli & Browne (1986) outline the role of day hospitals as the rehabilitation and promotion of function, promotion of socialisation and peer interaction and support for carers. Again, both individual and group treatment is provided within a multidisciplinary setting. Team members may include doctor, nursing staff, occupational therapist, physiotherapist, creative arts therapists and psychologist. Treatment may also be carried out in the person's own home or in other community environments. Day hospitals may be situated alongside ward areas or may be community based. Access to diagnostic facilities such as radiography and phlebotomy services is important.

SIGNIFICANT DISORDERS

Depression: the undetected illness

In clinical depression there is a sustained mood of sadness or grief which extends beyond normal experience. There have been various classifications of depression including mild and severe, neurotic and psychotic, endogenous and reactive and unipolar and bipolar. The variety of these classifications highlights the problems of categorising the experience of a particular client. However, understanding the characteristics of a depressive illness are important in planning occupational therapy.

Depression occurs throughout life and continues to be frequent well into old age. This may be a reoccurrence of unipolar (depression alone) or bipolar (depression and hypomania) type, or depression with more neurotic or reactive features. The prevalence of depression in elderly people in the community is approximately 10%, while most studies suggest that the prevalence of depression in elderly inpatients on non-psychiatric wards is considerably higher. In both community and inpatient settings a large proportion of sufferers are either undiagnosed or not receiving treatment. Freeling (1993) comments that this may be due to a failure of recognition of the illness by GPs and suggests that the routine screening of the over-75s by GPs be used to assess for the illness.

Depression has particular characteristics in its presentation in old age which make it more difficult to recognise. The client often presents with somatic features rather than with low mood. In addition, physical illnesses present in old age may mask depressive features. Some elderly people may not possess the language to articulate depressive symptoms due to cultural features. For example, there is no vernacular expression for depression in many eastern cultures.

Depression in elderly people may be due to environmental features associated with loss. Loss of job, status, financial security, close relationships, roles, home environment, bereavement and other life events are common in old age. Although elderly people respond well to treatment a significant minority are prone to relapse, the consequences of which can be serious leading to prolonged hospitalisation or even suicide.

A recent advance in the treatment of depression has been the introduction of the serotonin specific reuptake inhibitor (SSRI) antidepressants. These have fewer side effects than other anti-depressants and are less likely to cause sedation. This makes them useful for people with concurrent physical illnesses.

Occupational therapy facilitates expression of feelings and explores issues of loss through the use of creative techniques. It may also aim to tackle some of the practical effects of depression such as poor concentration and difficulty in decision making or problem solving. Occupational therapy will promote self-esteem and encourage the re-establishment of previous occupation and roles. Treatment programmes need to acknowledge the importance of maintenance of function, especially for those clients prone to relapse. Ong et al (1987) showed that relapse could be signi-ficantly reduced, over a period of 1 year, by a support group for depressed elderly people. This study is being extended to involve the relatives or carers of depressed people.

Alzheimer's disease: taking up a label

The term 'senile dementia' has been supplanted in the last 15 years by an extension of the concept of Alzheimer's disease to include those dementias arising after the age of 65 which share the same neuropathology as the presenile form. In 1977, the Medical Research Council produced a report entitled 'Senile and Presenile Dementia', which concluded that these disorders were now proper concerns for the scientific community (Lishman 1977).

What difference did this make? The notion that senile dementia was the same as being senile, that is old, fed ageist attitudes. It contributed to the view of elderly medicine and old age psychiatry as the Cinderellas of medicine. Those working in those specialities sometimes felt isolated and their skill in assessment and manage-ment was not recognised.

'Alzheimer made an honest woman of senile dementia by giving her a name. Instead of merely having aged disgracefully or lived too long, the demented elderly were acknowledged to be suffering from a disease' (Pitt 1990).

Concern about the proportion of the elderly world-wide who were suffering from the disease increased and hence the 'rising tide' became more public. Some public money was allocated to research and, once senile dementia was acknowledged as a disease and given a name, that name became available to carers. Alzheimer disease societies were set up by carers themselves, and their members have campaigned, heightened political awareness, raised money, spread knowledge and supported each other.

Accurate and early diagnosis of a dementing illness is vital. Again, a specialist service will ensure that an accurate history is obtained, a full medical examination is done and an objective cognitive assessment is performed. Scans such as computed tomography and magnetic resonance imaging are increasingly performed in order to confirm the disease process. The presentation and course of other forms of dementia vary and so increasingly specific diseases such as multi-infarct dementia or Lewey body disease are identified.

Occupational therapy aims to maintain functional ability for as long as possible whilst educating and supporting carers. Relatives and some clients will need opportunity to discuss the implications of the diagnosis and have their fears and worries acknowledged. Hereditary factors, for example, are often a particular concern. Occupational therapists can advise on the management of the disease in the home and give help in devising strategies to improve safety for features such as wandering.

Accurate functional assessments should be carried out at intervals in order to establish exactly what clients are still able to do for themselves and what areas of function are lost. This information is vital in arranging care in the community. Clients may need advice about driving and coping with risk. Memory aids may be suggested and consideration given to reinforcing routine. Legal advice is also important and clients may need to consider arranging an enduring power of attorney or appointing an advocate. Adaptation of the home environment may be necessary to improve safety or to maintain independence. This needs to be undertaken skilfully as changes in the environment can be disruptive to a person with Alzheimer's disease and can lead to further disorientation and loss of function.

Regular support for carers of people with dementia is important. Respite care should be available on a day basis and also to provide longer breaks. The prevalence of depression in informal care givers ranges from 30 to 50% (Butler & Madeley 1995). Carers find behavioural changes associated with the illness difficult to cope with, while communication difficulties such as receptive and expressive dysphasia make the relationship unrewarding and one-sided.

Anxiety states and phobias

Anxiety states and, to a lesser degree, phobic anxieties are common in elderly people. This is in spite of the fact that, based on referral rates, a myth existed that the incidence of neuroses declined with age. What was being observed was the result of elderly people failing to consult their doctor about neurotic problems and GPs not referring people to psychiatrists. In fact, after reaching a plateau in middle life, the incidence of neurosis starts to rise again with old age (Whitehead 1985).

Anxiety is a normal and essential part of human experience. In normal doses it increases a person's awareness, sharpens reactions and assists in avoiding danger. It is only when the degree of anxiety is excessive, or is triggered by inappropriate stimuli that it becomes damaging and disabling.

Older people may develop abnormal anxieties for a variety of reasons, ranging from a learned response to social situations present over many years, to a manifestation of alarm at the possibility of losing the family home. Severe anxiety can disturb the memory and take away the ability to carry out normal, relatively simple activities of daily living. In a younger person it is unlikely that such severe anxiety will be mistaken for the symptoms of Alzheimer's disease, but this may well be the case for an elderly person. Anxiety produces many somatic symptoms due to the physiological changes in the body as a result of the 'fight or flight' reaction. Rather than complaining of anxiety, the elderly person may well present with a physical problem such as breathlessness, unsteadiness, chest pain and fear of heart disease, abdominal pain and fears of cancer. The elderly person may also have an underlying depression as anxiety may lead to isolation and loneliness.

In phobic anxiety the factor which produces anxiety and fear is a specific situation or object which does not usually provoke anxiety in general. Some elderly people have had phobic anxieties for many years and may seek help for the first time in old age. Other phobias may have their onset in old age. A common phobia to occur for the first time in old age is the fear of falling. This may not be recognised as a true phobia due to social expectations of elderly people. Fear of falling may be associated with a person having had a fall or it may occur independently. Such a phobia can be very disruptive and lead to a person becoming housebound and isolated. Ironically, a fear of falling may exist alongside associated mobility problems and other conditions which may lead a person to be prone to falls.

Occupational therapy is effective in reducing anxiety and in teaching alternative coping strategies. As in other areas of old age psychiatry, the client may have been experiencing the problem for a number of years and so the treatment programme needs to be specific and realistic. This is not to suggest that long-standing difficulties may not be treated. However, it is important to explore with the client how the illness or problem is viewed by the client and his or her family or carer. A particular difficulty may be framed by the client in complex ways which become part of the family structure or folklore. To intervene through occupational therapy may upset the balance of loss and gain that the illness invokes and therefore treatment should be negotiated.

The occupational therapist will assess the client, obtaining as much information as possible about the onset and nature of anxiety, what triggers it and how it presents. It will be important to assess levels of anxiety within the client's occupational performance and explore the way in which the anxiety is framed by the client and the relevant family members. The client may have developed skill deficits through the avoidance of certain anxiety-provoking situations. For example, a client had not used public transport for a number of years and consequently was unable to use the automatic ticket machines which had been installed in buses. Such deficits should be identified in order to design a programme to teach new skills.

Education about anxiety is important as many clients do not realise that anxiety is normal. Information should be presented in a clear format that will be easy to remember, as it is important that learning is carried over into the anxiety-provoking situation. There are a variety of attractive materials available including workbooks, posters, videos and tapes. This subject is explored more fully in Chapter 9.

The occupational therapy programme will teach the use of effective relaxation techniques. Again it is vital that having learned a new skill this is carried over into the client's own environment. 'Anxiety management' either individually or in a group setting is an effective method of promoting new coping strategies and encouraging the re-establishment of roles and routines that have been interrupted.

ISSUES IN INTERVENTION
Techniques in occupational therapy

The list in Box 3.1 provides, for reference purposes, a reminder of approaches which may be included within a programme of occupational therapy. Each, in the broader contexts of therapy, is described either elsewhere in this volume or is well documented in other professional texts. Those which have not been developed specifically to meet the needs of elderly people may need to be adapted or used with sensitivity to the particular set of problems or priorities identified.

Box 3.1

Anxiety management	Life review
Relaxation training	Counselling
Problem solving	Assertiveness training
Cognitive approaches	Leisure activities
Reality of orientation	Adaptation of environment
Validation therapy	Communication work
Reminiscence therapy	Creative expression
Functional work	Domestic skills
Education	Behavioural approaches

This reminder is not, of course, exhaustive. Occupational therapists faced by the variety of challenges posed by this age group will need to draw on their full repertoire of physical, psychological and social skills.

Decision making and consent

It is a basic common law principle that a person's body is inviolate and that any intentional touching of it without consent is a trespass. Thus any medical procedure involving touch performed without consent is, in legal terms, a civil wrong. This rule has been modified by what is termed the doctrine of necessity. Necessity provides a justification for intervention, such as emergency treatment, for which consent cannot be obtained.

Occupational therapists should be clear that they need to obtain consent from a client for any intervention, however straightforward it might seem. Giving consent to treatment means that the person should be fully and properly informed about the suggested procedure, its risks and the consequences of refusing it. For consent to be valid, it is important to establish that the client understands in broad terms what is involved. This may take time and therefore opportunities to give consent should be repeated, particularly for clients with short-term memory problems. It is not acceptable to assume consent is given if a person does not object to treatment—opportunity must be given for the person to object. The caring relationship places the client in a very unequal position where the professional holds the power. Whilst many clients feel grateful to their carer or practitioner and feel unable to question a procedure, others feel that to question a procedure will jeopardise their future treatment. Too often medical language styles simply do not allow the space for the client to participate in the decision-making process.

An important issue is the question of how to proceed if a person is incapable of giving consent to treatment. A legal incapacity arises whenever the law provides that a person is incapable of taking a particular decision or engaging in a particular transaction. Under law, the general approach has been that it is presumed that the person is capable unless proved otherwise, and capacity is judged in relation to the particular decision to be made at that particular time. Incapacity to make a decision may be due to a variety of causes, some of them due to mental health problems. The Mental Health Act 1983 is very specific in the scope it allows for using its powers to give compulsory treatment or detention.

The policy of community care has resulted in more people with a mental health problem being cared for in the community rather than an institution. The benefits of living as normal a life as possible are recognised as being preferable to the restrictions of an institution. Life in the community does, however, make people with these difficulties more vulnerable and more likely targets for abuse or exploitation. In responding to this there is a very real danger that such people have their dignity stripped away through overprotection by their carers. What must be considered is that the risk of institutionalisation may be much greater than the risk of occasionally being open to making an unwise decision. Living in the community means being free to experience normal risks and sometimes make mistakes. However, the supervision register, part of the care programme approach, exists in order to ensure that those people at most risk or posing a risk to others receive the appropriate support and treatment.

For those people unable to make an informed decision, the doctrine of necessity may be used to determine what treatment may be administered without the person's consent. This is not always helpful as some procedures are desirable rather than necessary. An alternative principle in law is that of best interests—that is, treatment may be given if it can be demonstrated that the procedure is in the client's best interests. The concept of what is or is not in someone's best interests is open to many interpretations, so how should a person's best interests be assessed?

Traditionally it has been medical staff who have decided what is in a person's best interests. Increasingly, however, family members or carers are involved in this decision making. To ensure good practice, a client should have an advocate appointed to look after his or her best interests. This is important, as family members may have an agenda which is different from or opposed to the that of the client. Although not yet implemented in some areas of practice, this was recommended by the Disabled Persons (Services, Consultation and Representation) Act 1986 and by the National Health Service and Community Care Act 1990.

Advocacy

Advocates may assist professionals in the important job of determining what is in the client's best interests but may also suggest what the client might have wanted had he or she been able to say. This is particularly valid in the case of a person with Alzheimer's disease who has previously had capacity and may have expressed opinions on the subject, or left evidence of what his or her wishes might be. In such a case it might be preferable to adopt the principle of substituted judgement, by which decisions are decided in the way the person would have acted.

For example, in order to achieve an individual's definition of a dignified death, some people are drawing up living wills. Whilst not yet a legal document in England, these set down beforehand a person's wishes regarding his or her treatment in the event of a serious illness. In order to address this important area of civil rights, Age Concern has drawn up a 'charter of rights to community care for older people'. The charter contains the following statement of purpose:

each older person has the right to a life which maintains personal independence, safeguards privacy, offers genuine and informed choices, provides opportunities to enjoy and contribute to society as fully as possible and meets his/her social, cultural and individual needs. If such an independent life involves a degree of risk which the older person accepts, the authority will respect such a wish and endeavour to support the individual wherever possible.

Elder abuse

Vulnerable adults do not have the long-established and detailed legislation that children have to protect their rights. There are no detailed investigative procedures to ensure that abuse can be identified and dealt with. In law, adults are considered independent and therefore able to protect their rights.

Although the prevalence of elder abuse remains unknown and difficult to determine, the most reliable US research suggests the figure of 4% (Godkin et al 1989). Health workers who have encountered cases of abuse, neglect or exploitation of elderly people find the ethical dilemmas posed in such situations the most difficult to resolve.

The central ethical dilemma is the right of an adult to self-determination versus the freedom of protection from violence or exploitation and the loss of dignity. Some elderly people who do experience abuse do not wish any action to be taken as the consequences of acknowledging the abuse are too great. The most frequent intervention in cases of abuse is the removal of the elderly person from the situation, often leading to the loss of a home, independence and reduced contact with family members. A similar dilemma exists when an elderly person refuses services or treatment and yet is clearly at risk. How far should professionals override personal autonomy to protect an at-risk individual?

Since the increase in awareness of child abuse in the 1960s social and health care workers have attempted to balance the need for protection of the child, the wishes of the child and parental rights and autonomy. This has been formalised in the Children Act 1989. In the case of an abused older person, however, the expectations of when and how intervention should take place have yet to be debated at a national level. This means that individual service providers have a responsibility for developing local policy and procedure for this important issue.

REFERENCES

Age Concern 1991 Old age abuse, lifting the lid. Age Concern, England
Arie T (ed) 1985 Recent advances in psychogeriatrics. Churchill Livingstone, Edinburgh
Butler J, Madeley P 1995 Depression in carers. Geriatric Medicine 25(2): 41–43
Children Act 1989 HMSO, London

Cirirelli V G, Browne E 1986 Psychological considerations in the day care of elderly people. In: Hanley I, Gilhooley M (eds) Psychological therapies for the elderly. Croom Helm, London

Department of Health 1990 Caring for people policy guidance. HMSO, London

Disabled Persons (Services, Consultation and Representation) Act 1986 HMSO, London

Freeling P 1993 Diagnosis and treatment of depression in general practice. British Journal of Psychiatry 163(20): 14–19

Godkin M A, Wolf R S, Pillemer K A 1989 A case comparison analysis of elder abuse and neglect. International Journal of Ageing and Human Development 28(3): 207–225

Health Advisory Service 1982 The rising tide: developing services for mental illness in old age. Department of Health Advisory Service, Sutton

Lishman W A (ed) 1977 Senile and presenile dementias. Medical Research Council, London

Mental Health Act 1983 HMSO, London

Neugarten B L 1970 The old and the young in modern societies. American Behavioural Scientist 14: 13–24

National Health Service and Community Care Act 1990 HMSO, London

Ong Y L, Martineau F, Lloyd C, Robbins I 1987 A support group for the depressed elderly. International Journal of Geriatric Psychiatry 2: 119–123

Pitt B 1990 Turning points: Alzheimer's disease. Geriatric Medicine 20(5): 19–20

Whitehead J A 1985 Recognising and treating anxiety state and phobia. Geriatric Medicine 15(2): 31–33

PART 2

Key concepts

PART CONTENTS

4

A humanistic perspective

Elizabeth Cracknell

There are two modes of knowing, those of argument and experience.

Roger Bacon, English monk and scholar, 1214–1292

INTRODUCTION

Human beings are constantly trying to make sense of the world, their experiences of it and their place within it. Experiences happen both within us, to us and around us and we struggle to interpret and give meaning to these events so that we understand what is happening to us. Past experience tells us that if we stand with a group of friends and watch a meeting between two strangers in the street, each of us will perceive the incident differently. Questioning would reveal that some information in the observers' descriptions would be common to all, whilst some would be different. However, the interpretations at the assumption level might be quite dissimilar, leading to different understandings and explanations. How does this happen? Objects in the world exist, and we take in knowledge of them in the form of raw data, such as sound and light waves, through the senses. We interpret the sensations and give them meaning; thereby we come to an understanding of our experience. It is the acceptance of the validity of people's own subjective experiences, wherein each person is unique, which is at the heart of humanistic psychology and differentiates it from other theoretical perspectives.

As an approach to the study of people, humanistic psychology includes a number of different theories, which are bound together by a particular view of people. Human beings are accepted as being responsible, free organisms who make choices and are not just responsive creatures without thought or feeling. The theory says that my understanding of what is happening to me is valid, even if it differs from that of other people, and as such, has to be accepted as real for me. If that be so, as I am the only person who knows what I understand, I am the best person to say what I need and explain my actions, not some outside observer. Although old, in the sense that the fundamental concerns of what it means to be human have been expressed through the ages in art, literature, philosophy and religion, it is a comparatively new school of thought in psychology and is strongly identified with the upsurge of the human potential movement in the United States of the 1960s and 1970s.

In the late nineteenth century, William James had advocated a psychology which recognised the wholeness and uniqueness of the individual; ideas which were emphasised in the 1930s by the personality theorists Goldstein, Allport, Maslow and Rollo May. However, not until the 1950s did humanistic psychology as a name exist, and, in spite of the similarity of name, it should not be confused with humanism. Abraham H Maslow (1908–1970) is often regarded as the founding father of current humanistic psychology for he published what is perhaps the first complete statement of this approach in his book, *Motivation and Personality*, in 1954; a classic of its time. Having decided on a name for the new person-focused psychology, Maslow and Anthony Sutich spent 3 years preparing the launch of the *Journal of Humanistic Psychology* in 1961.

The rise of the 'third force' of humanistic psychology immediately challenged other theories in psychology, for the assumptions upon which it is based contrast sharply with other branches of psychology. It is not deterministic as is psychoanalysis, for it does not assume that the individual is in the hapless grip of unconscious forces; neither is it mechanistic, as is behaviourism, assuming that the individual is like a machine and only works when the button is pushed. In humanistic psychology the individual is a growing, developing, creating creature, with a capacity and freedom to make choices and take full self-responsibility. It is an optimistic view of human nature grounded in a belief that people are essentially good, and are motivated by an innate force driving them toward the goal of 'actualisation'. In other words, we human beings move and function in ways that enable us to grow, change and expand our potential being with which we are born. What a challenge to an exciting journey of life. Our sense of 'well-being' depends upon the way we direct the motivational forces, the choices we make as each of us moves to enhance our being.

A basic tenet is that the individual always responds to events as a whole organism; consequently it is not possible to study small isolated elements of behaviour, for every part of one's being influences other aspects. To study people within the parameters of this framework means selecting carefully an appropriate research method which is compatible with the basic philosophy. Rowan (1988), in his interesting text on humanistic psychology, writes: 'It is a whole new way of looking at psychological science. It is a way of doing science which includes love, involvement and spontaneity, instead of systematically excluding them' (p. 3).

In this chapter we will look at some of the roots of humanistic psychology and at the contributions made by two major figures in this field, Abraham Maslow and Carl Rogers. We will then look at the current scene in humanistic psychology and some of the constraints which limit the expression of these ideas in society today.

THE ORIGINS OF HUMANISTIC PSYCHOLOGY

Psychological theories rarely appear as complete entities; neither are they static bodies of knowledge. Theories evolve through a process of dialectic; that is, the truth of a theory is disputed and discussed and subsequently the theory evolves. All theories are strongly influenced by other ideas that abound at the time of their formulation, and humanistic theories are particularly interesting as they have roots anchored both in eastern and western thinking. Rowan (1988) traces the strands from their origins and describes how they entwined to become humanistic psychology as we know it today. Three distinct groups of ideas, phenomenology, existentialism and self theories as evident in groups and small group work, are found within this perspective and we shall have a look at each one.

The philosophy of the humanistic approach has extended beyond the bounds of psychology to other disciplines. The client-centred theories which arose from counselling and psychotherapy grew into person-centred psychology as it influenced the thinking of people in education, clinical and social psychology, counselling and psychotherapy, management and occupational therapy. Mearns & Thorne (1988) show how in the 1980s the ideas which stem from this school of thought extended to cross-cultural communication and international peace work.

Phenomenology

Phenomenology is the theory of 'phenomena' derived from the Greek word *phainomenon* (plural: *phainomena*) and literally means 'appearances'. In philosophy 'phenomena' means the appearances of things, in contrast with the things as they really are. Immanuel Kant (1724–1804) argued that it was not possible for human beings to know the true nature of reality; it is only known to us through our senses as we interpret events. Consequently we can only know the world as it appears to us to be; the phainomena. Through experience we live in a phenomenal world. That raises a question of what is really out there and how real is it for each person. Edmund Husserl (1859–1938), the German philosopher, adopted the term for his method of enquiry, the phenomenological method, wherein he attempted to investigate how human beings present reality to their own consciousness. He believed that the subjective reality of an individual, however distorted or erroneous, is of greater value than the objective reality. He was particularly interested in how the mind translates the raw stimuli which bombard the senses as they arrive from the real world to be translated into a meaningful object-based reality in consciousness. A process he called 'intentionality'.

The significance of Husserl's enquiry can be recognised if we reflect upon what factors influence our behaviour. Knowledge of the world enters our consciousness as raw data through our senses. The sensations we receive are perceived, that is they are organised and interpreted, in order for them to become part of our consciousness. However, our interpretations are influenced by such things as our beliefs, values, attitudes, personal disposition and interests; indeed all aspects of our being. We hear this demonstrated daily in the political life of the country. Whenever we listen to politicians discussing new ideas, such as educational reform, we hear people from different parties taking such different lines on the issue that one would hardly recognise that they are talking about the same thing. Each person's response is coloured by the values and political views that he or she holds, which differ to such a degree that, at times, it would appear that politicians have great difficulty in communicating with each other. Politicians from different parties do not live in the same phenomenal world and events are interpreted from within dissimilar perceptual frameworks. As our interpretations are the basis for thoughts and actions, varying opinions are expressed and behaviour will most likely accord with those views.

Here is an example on a simpler, personal level. When shopping in town the other day I saw a familiar figure of a friend ahead of me in the street. I had not seen her for months so hurried to catch up with her. I put out my hand and touched her on the shoulder and said, 'Hello Mary'. She turned; it was not Mary. I had acted upon information which I had misperceived and felt embarrassed and foolish, for I had made a mistake. From my point of view, my behaviour was rational and understandable for it was based upon my perceptions of events. Misperceptions, which occur to all of us, are usually rectified, but if there is a large distortion of external reality through interpretation, behaviour can appear to others to be foolhardy or even bizarre.

We live in a phenomenal world, for our conclusions are based upon a number of psychological and social factors, and are thereby relative. That is hard for us to accept and we usually behave as if our understandings are certain, but of course they are not. Some philosophers argue that it is not possible to know the real world at all. Rogers (1959, p. 194) wrote 'Man essentially lives in his own personal and subjective world, and even his most objective functioning in science, mathematics and the like, is the result of subjective purpose and subjective choice'. Spinelli (1989) filled a gap in the literature with *The Interpreted World*, in which he explores phenomenal psychology and its philosophical connections. In it he emphasises that, although phenomenology stresses the uniquenesses and differences between individuals, that does not minimise the shared features of human experience. Phenomenological psychology redresses the balance in a world which has been dominated by a study of the commonalities of being human.

In the summer of 1993, I heard a different expression of these ideas in a series of lectures by Professor John Hull of Birmingham University. His thesis was that, knowing occurs bodily, not just through the head, but through the whole of the body, and as such the phenomenal world of men is different from that of women, that of able-bodied people is different from that of disabled people, a child's phenomenal world is different from that of the adult and that of the rich man from that of the poor. For each person it is unique. As Professor Hull is blind, the lectures had a very powerful impact upon all the listeners present; his world is very different from ours.

The influence of existentialism

It is impossible to explain all the complexities of this body of thought as it is amorphous and shifts in emphasis as it developed in different directions. It was Martin Heidegger (1889–1976), who worked with Husserl in the 1920s and later taught philosophy, who first formulated the origins of existential thought. Existentialist philosophers emphasise the contrast between human existence and that of the rest of the world, the natural objects. People are differentiated from their material surroundings and other animals by consciousness and the freedom to make choices through which they can transcend their biological constraints. This particular view of being, Heidegger called Dasein, literally 'being there'; more often loosely interpreted as 'being in the world'. It is not a happy condition of being, for it is characterised by an anxious awareness of the future and of impending death, i.e. the cessation of being. Within this gloomy state of affairs we can choose the meanings that we give to our experiences. By the decisions we make, we take part in our own creation or limit it depending upon the choices we make. We are not endowed with character and goals but choose them in the way we live and move towards our destiny. Existentialists believe that we are creatures who are constantly searching for meaning and purpose in life, and every person has to discover this for him- or herself.

In his search for meaning in life, Heidegger conceptualised two styles of being: inauthentic and authentic existence. As in-authentic beings, we are conformist and conventional and fail to recognise our own being in relation to the world. We avoid facing the temporal nature of our being and live according to the prevailing norms of the society in which we live. We fail to exercise the freedom that we have, responding to life's experiences from a reactive and thereby irresponsible position. On the other hand, as authentic beings we are able to confront the knowledge of death as an event of life, the ultimate of human existence, and live with a knowledge that individuality is a set of potentialities, not a static state of being. We live with an independence of thought and action as we conceive the world as available for human activity. As a result of our decisions, we feel in charge of ourselves in our activity in the world. Consequently we become more integrated in the world, more open and alive in 'being in the world'. Failure to achieve this interrelatedness in the world through meaningful relationships may result in loneliness, isolation, hopelessness and despair.

Ideas grounded in existentialism have spread to many disciplines over the last 50 years. They are to be found in theological writings of Martin Buber and Paul Tillich; in psychoanalytical thinking of Ludwig Binswanger, Medard Boss and Erich Fromm; in the literature of Jean Paul Sartre and Albert Camus; and in British psychiatry, through the thinking of Ronald Laing.

The influence of 'groups'

The third strand of humanistic psychology is perhaps the one that is seen as having a particular relevance to occupational therapists as so often we use group methods to treat individual people. However, we need to be aware of the other two strands of this approach if we are to really understand group work and the powerful impact it can have on individual group members. The interest in the study of groups began with the work of Kurt Lewin (1890–1947), a social psychologist, who revolutionised this field with his work showing that complex social phenomena could be studied using experimental methods. His ideas of behaviour being a function of the person and the environment as that person perceives it gave rise to many general theoretical concepts to be found in social psychology today. Lewin's experiences in Nazi Germany left him with a strong desire to find ways of using groups to help participants develop more democratic approaches to the exercise of leadership. At the Massachusetts Institute of Technology in the 1940s, Lewin established groups for managers and executives from large organisations to help them develop democratic attitudes and be more sensitive to the dynamics of interpersonal relationships at work. He coined the term 'group dynamics' to describe these processes.

In 1946, trainees on a particular course asked to sit in on an evening meeting between trainers and observers. Such a request had never been made before and must have caused anxiety in everyone involved. The resulting discussion of trainees, trainers and observers went on well into the night with emotions at times running high, almost to the point of explosion as views were expressed freely and openly. For the first time in group work, honest feedback had occurred. The members found it to be such an exciting, valuable learning experience, that even though it was at times a painful process, they requested further involvement in their own course. The inclusion of feedback on these courses continued from then on and their success led to the founding of the National Training Laboratories in 1947. Training in human relations skills by means of 'T-groups' where 'T' stands for 'training' had demonstrated that democratic leadership was effective in western society, for it reduced autocracy, rigidity and the hierarchical nature of structures and enabled people in organisations to be more positive and less resentful. Even though these effects have been clearly demonstrated, there is still a reluctance in organisations to adopt these approaches.

At the same time as Lewin was embarking upon his study of groups, Carl Rogers was experimenting in the use of groups for training graduate students in counselling at the University of Chicago. His style of administering the Counselling Centre arose directly from his own philosophy embodied in his counselling practice and writings. His students were all very able, for they were all well qualified academically, but he felt that an approach which involved the participants experimentally would be more appropriate. Participants met in an intensive group experience for several hours a day to study their attitudes, emotional behaviour and the relationships which they established with each other. The experiences together often led beyond the improvement of communication and personal skills to personal development and growth. Later in California, building on previous experience, Rogers worked with groups for people who were not following formal education, but wanted experiences in a group which would encourage personal growth. Rogers' style of working in a group grew from his own client-centred approach in individual therapy. The groups were relatively unstructured, for participants were able to choose their own goals, whilst the role of the group leader was to create a climate of safety which facilitated members in the expression of their thoughts and feelings as they were then experiencing them in relation to others in the group. In this safe climate, trust developed as members were able to be authentic, that is express their true feelings of appreciation, anxiety, irritation and love so that individuals become more accepting of themselves and others. Rogers called his groups, basic encounter groups. From 1961, when the Esalen Institute was founded, encounter groups developed slightly differently, incorporating techniques of human potential such as psychodrama, meditation and Gestalt work.

The confluence of ideas from the work of Lewin and Rogers manifested itself in the development of the human potential movement through the 1960s, which seemed to explode in the 1970s. The surge of these ideas served to promote an awareness of others and the growth of interactional skills in each individual group member. Experience is shared and reflected upon together, facilitating a greater confidence, spontaneity and freedom to be oneself.

In occupational therapy, creative expressive work may be a direct application of the principles of humanistic psychology, whether it be as education or therapy. If, as a member of a trusting group, I paint my first remembered embarrassing experience and share my experience of that event with other members, it is my thoughts, feelings and subjective reality which is of value, not the perceptions of others. I may respond to some ideas that other group members offer me and learn from them, but in humanistic psychology, the client knows best. By listening to me, other members will have a greater understanding of my inner world; I do not need an outsider to interpret it for me but I do need others to listen and accept what I say.

Similarly, in individual work, when I am working with a client who has limited function due to rheumatoid arthritis, and I try to understand her world view and her treatment goals, I am adopting a person-centred approach. I do not say, 'This is what you need, let's go for it.' I talk to her so that I may understand what her priorities are, and these will depend upon her personal perspective. To be of value to her, treatment has to be related to her perception of the world and her place in it. Her experience provides part of the basis for treatment and, by being involved in the process, she is making decisions on her own behalf. In humanistic terms she is encouraged in the process of enhancing her own being and developing her own potential.

Maslow takes a broad view of human nature and links

personality with motivation. He suggests that we become the people we are as a result of how our basic needs are met in life. It is his theory we go on to next.

THE CONTRIBUTION OF ABRAHAM MASLOW

Many personality psychologists developed theoretical approaches which are humanistic in orientation, among them Erich Fromm, Gordon Allport and Carl Rogers. Abraham Maslow (1908–1970), with his holistic–dynamic theory of personality, includes most of the major concepts that these theorists have in common. In his early years, Abraham Maslow was attracted to behaviourism and was undoubtedly influenced by psychoanalysis, but his questioning and 'intuitive conviction' led him down new avenues. He writes that his explorations of new ideas created in him great anxiety; nevertheless it did not deter him from producing very positive results.

In 1954, Maslow's *Motivation and Personality* presented the first complete statement of the new humanistic psychology. In the 1970 edition, he wrote that he 'attempted to enlarge our conception of the human personality by reaching into the "higher" levels of human nature'. Similar ideas expressed by Maslow in *Towards a Psychology of Being* (1968) had a profound effect upon me when I first read it, for it spoke to me in a way which resounded with my own experiences. For Maslow, all aspects of our beings are interrelated and all affect each other; hence the whole healthy person was the subject of his studies. Maslow did not accept as valid the study of discrete parts of the organism such as behaviour or the psychodynamics. Nor did he focus on people who showed disturbed or maladjusted behaviours, but on people who appeared to him to function well and cope with life. One of his quests was to discover what motivates ordinary people like us throughout life and on what basis do we choose our options.

From his studies of both normal and exceptional people—those he considered to be 'self-actualising'—he found that they had particular characteristics in common. His investigations revealed that these people seemed 'to be fulfilling themselves and doing the best they are capable of doing' (Maslow 1970, p. 150). Maslow's new philosophy of the person comprised a holistic view of people wherein each individual is unique and can only be studied as a dynamic whole. He promoted a positive, more hopeful and encouraging view of people, based upon a belief that human nature is not intrinsically evil but, in essence, neutral or good. It was not the essence of feelings such as anger and fear which was evil although he recognised that the power of them could lead to evil behaviour. Maslow wrote that as human beings we have distinctive features such as self-awareness, creativity and compassion, which set us apart from other organisms. He believed that each person has an innate capacity for growth and development, and that emotional maturity means realising one's inherent potential and accepting one's individuality and aloneness.

Maslow's theory of motivation consists of a hierarchical system of needs and it is the drive to fulfil these physical and psychological sets of needs which directs our behaviour. Our subsequent actions in turn contribute to the growth of our individual inherent potential. This inner force pushes us towards self-actualisation, the process of developing the full stature of which we are capable.

The motivational hierarchy of needs

Maslow studied healthy people over a 2-year period as they went about their daily business. He observed people at work, solving problems, buying insurance, running competitively, purchasing goods and in pursuit of other common daily activities. He spent some time studying the biographies of great people such as Abraham Lincoln and Albert Schweitzer. He also studied a group of people who, on the basis of their achievements in life, seemed to merit being described as self-actualisers. He noted that patterns emerged in behaviour which showed that, at times, different needs tended to dominate behaviour. His observations led to the proposal that motives could be categorised in a hierarchical way and, only if the needs of the lower category were satisfied, would the needs of the higher levels emerge and determine behaviour. From a developmental point of view, lower level needs manifest themselves earlier in life than do higher level needs and must be attended to before higher level needs emerge. Another aspect of needs is that the higher the level of needs the greater the differentiation of human beings from other elements of nature, i.e. plants and animals.

Maslow devised a hierarchy of five distinct levels of need which emerge in a set order. He described the needs of levels 1 to 4 as 'deficiency' needs, as they were those which maintained the individual, whilst the needs of level 5 he regarded as higher order growth needs, alternatively referred to as self-actualising needs, or 'metaneeds'. Higher needs are long-term needs and always active, unlike the deficiency needs which are transitory and can be satisfied fairly quickly, even if only temporarily. In his view we are all motivated by these needs, and different ones may emerge at different times depending upon our circumstances.

The physiological needs

Physiological needs are those related to survival and maintenance of the body. Maslow describes these needs as the most important, for if a person lacks the basic necessities of life the physiological needs of hunger, thirst, warmth, shelter and sleep will motivate behaviour. Such is the plight of people suffering from famine in Somalia and Ethiopia and indeed a growing number of young people on the streets in London. The need for food to live, to satisfy hunger, dominates their lives and, if this desperate need is not met, death ensues. If food, water and shelter are found and the basic needs are satisfied at an acceptable level, and for most of us in this society they are met, then the next group of needs appears and motivates behaviour. An exception to this is the need for sexual satisfaction, for we human beings can live a continent life without this being detrimental to our state of being.

Safety needs

Safety needs are concerned with our security from physical danger, the avoidance of pain and the maintenance of psychological security. Maslow includes protection, and freedom from anxiety and chaos—a need for structure and law. In a well-organised stable society our safety needs are generally well met so they will not become active motivators. However, at the time of recession, a woman threatened with redundancy is in no physical danger but is psychologically endangered, for the future is extremely uncertain. The security needs motivate her actions for they will dominate her life, and the anxiety which surrounds her as a result of the position in which she finds herself will direct her behaviour to change the situation. She will attempt to hang on to her present position, combat the redundancy and at the same time look for another job. All other interests and activities will be less important and may for a time disappear until the safety needs have been satisfied. Similarly, a child who lives in an environment with no consistent rules and boundaries will not feel secure and will be unable to satisfy the inner needs at this level. As a result, behaviour will be directed to finding greater security, which may not be in a way that is understood by parents and will thereby create misunderstandings and difficulties.

Belongingness and love needs

When the physiological and safety needs are satisfied our needs for love and affection become predominant. These include our needs of intimacy, the receiving and acceptance of trust, affection, and the pleasure we have with each other. When these needs emerge, we become very aware of the absence of friends and family and will seek people out in order to meet these needs. Contact with family, colleagues and friends at work or in leisure, are natural ways of satisfying the needs of belongingness and love. However, many people in our society do not interact daily with people in a way which meets their belonging needs, for they may live alone, away from family and friends. For a society to survive and be healthy, Maslow writes that the belongingness and love needs must be met. Some psychologists believe that the expansion of the group movement in the 1970s and 80s may be partly due to the unmet needs for intimate relationships of people who live in a mobile society where traditional groups are scattered or broken. Sex may be an element of these love needs, as it is usually associated with the giving and receiving of love, but it can be studied as a purely physiological need.

The esteem needs

Maslow recognised the powerful need we all have to feel good about ourselves. We need a high evaluation of ourselves. He believed that we need to esteem and regard ourselves well and we need the esteem of others. There is a strong desire for achievement, for meeting the challenge of mastering the environment, for competence and confidence to cope with the world. From other people the individual needs recognition, regard, prestige, affirmation and appreciation, which contribute to a growth of confidence, strength and feelings of self-worth. The thwarting of these needs leads to feelings of inferiority and helplessness. The most healthy self-esteem is based upon respect from others which is earned, rather than fame or unwarranted adulation. These four groups of 'deficiency need' associated with survival have to be satisfied before the metaneeds associated with actualisation become salient.

Self-actualisation needs

In August 1993, I watched Linford Christie on television run the 100 metres sprint and win a gold medal in the world athletic championships. He was not running in the race as a way of surviving or meeting his deficiency needs. He had trained hard and had developed his physical potential and become one of the best athletes in the world. According to the hierarchy of needs, Christie's physical and psychological needs have all been met. His esteem and belonging needs are satisfied, for his motivation is very different from that which drives a person who is functioning as a result of some unmet deficiency need. He is realising some of his being needs, those of physical prowess wherein he pushes ever further his boundaries of being. In Maslow's thinking, the goal of healthy living is self-actualisation, the process whereby individuals develop fully and become what they are potentially able to become. Three groups of needs are regarded as higher needs and in current texts are often separated, although in Maslow's own thinking they were interrelated. Firstly, the cognitive needs of needing to know. We need to understand and explore what is going on in the world. Secondly, our aesthetic needs which are concerned with the appreciation of symmetry, order, truth, goodness and beauty, and finally those needs concerned with the fulfilment and realisation of self. These levels of need are the motivational forces for our behaviour and, although every person has the capacity for self-actualisation, few people achieve it because lower needs are not satisfied in a way which enables the higher needs to become active.

Some characteristics of self-actualising people

Maslow observed that there were common features in those people whom he regarded as having realised their potential. He wrote that these people are likely to have:

- superior perception of reality which is not distorted by personal wants and needs

- a realism in their acceptance of themselves, their strengths and weaknesses, and of others and the natural world
- a greater spontaneity of expression, thought and behaviour
- a problem-solving approach to life rather than self-preoccupation
- a need for privacy, and their higher autonomy means less dependence on others
- a vivid appreciation of things around them
- a spirituality, though not necessarily in the formal religious sense; they may have 'peak experiences' when they feel ecstatically powerful, transcendent and yet at one with the world
- intimacy of a deep nature with a few well-chosen friends
- democratic values; they are open and spontaneous with others whoever they are
- a recognition of the difference between ends and means
- a sense of humour which is not hostile but more philosophical
- a capacity for humour and creativity
- a certain non-conformity, resisting cultural pressures.

A rather daunting list and Maslow considered that few people ever achieved such maturity. He did find, however, that some of his subjects had what he called mystical or spiritual experiences, states of extreme joy and pleasure, expressed bodily with perhaps a lump in the throat, tears in the eyes, prickles, a wish to shout. Such an experience was rare for it may have happened only once or twice in a lifetime. Maslow called these 'peak' experiences and explained them as evidence that people did have untapped resources and he believed that such experiences revealed aspects of reality which are normally hidden.

Maslow's theory of motivation has been applied in many fields but is particularly helpful in the understanding of individuals within large organisations. We can adopt this perspective when we are trying to understand our own behaviour as employees in large bureaucratic organisations as well as the behaviour of clients. The theory provides a framework for assessing a person's needs which includes not just satisfying the deficiency needs but also the higher metaneeds which are part of a person's whole being. A society which is well structured will not just provide food and shelter for its people, but also enable them to develop their potential capacity, thereby adding an unrealised richness and vitality to the whole community.

THE CONTRIBUTION OF CARL ROGERS

Carl Rogers' (1902–1987) contribution to humanistic psychology arises from his work as a therapist. Rogers was born into a fairly strict religious family in Chicago, a fact which he described later in life as 'rather burdensome'. In his early years he was interested in the biological sciences and the scientific grounding he gained was invaluable to him. He left school to enter the Union Theological Seminary of New York City with the intention of becoming a priest but did not stay long, moving to Columbia University to read psychology where he was strongly influenced by the philosopher, John Dewey (1859–1952). His subsequent clinical studies, teaching and researches created in him a growing interest in personality and psychotherapy. In his initial clinical work he was exposed to Freudian thought but found himself much more in sympathy with theorists who emphasised the importance of 'the self' as a concept influencing behaviour. Rogers' writings, which continued throughout his life, are regarded as the most articulate, comprehensive and systematic, in the humanistic psychology tradition.

Rogers presented his first formulation of this theory as an approach to therapy in *Client Centred Therapy* (1951) and a celebration of 50 years of the person-centred approach was marked by a special edition of *Person-Centred Review* in 1990. However, Rogers free thinking was applied in many other fields as well as psychology. *Freedom to Learn* (1969) was thoroughly revised as *Freedom to Learn for the 80s* (1983) as his contribution to education. His involvement in the encounter movement resulted in his book *Encounter Groups* (1970), whilst in the 1970s he became increasingly interested in broader social and political issues. Many of his thoughts were published in a collection of papers *A Way of Being* (1980). In his later years Rogers became involved in peace studies, international relations and running workshops on the person-centred approach around the world.

Theoretical rationale

Rogerian theory, like others within this school of thought, proposes that the organism (the whole person) is a holistic entity motivated to maintain and enhance itself. This motivating drive energises behaviour in the direction of the full development of the inherent potentialities of the person. It is a way of living which leads to greater differentiation and integration as the individual moves towards becoming a 'fully functioning' person. As this process progresses, greater independence develops and freedom of expression grows. 'Fully functioning' is the title of the last chapter of Rogers' revised edition of *Freedom to Learn* (1983). Rogers believed that we human beings, have within us great capacities for choice, virtue, self-understanding and for changing our self-concepts, attitudes and behaviours. In particular climates these inner resources, which may be unknown to us, can be tapped and released and we are thereby able to develop and change. It is this belief that gives rise to my statement to students that they have greater resources than they think they have, and it is our responsibility as teachers, to create a climate in which they can get in touch with, and develop these capacities. But what does this all mean?

The self

In his clinical work, Rogers found that people interpreted and evaluated their experiences in relation to a 'self-concept'. He observed that most clients were motivated in a direction of growth and positive change. As a result of these experiences, the concept of 'self' as part of the whole organism became central to Rogers' theory of personality. He believed we all carry within us a concept of self which encompasses the organised set or pattern of perceptions, feelings, attitudes and values which makes us unique beings. It comprises both the 'I' and the 'me' aspects of self and refers to the conscious sense of who we are as people. To put it in everyday words, although we all deceive ourselves to some extent, we can describe ourselves to some degree, say who we believe we are. I can also be subject to myself. When I say I am proud of myself, there is in that statement a recognition of the I and the me components of self. It encompasses our own subjective thoughts and feelings about ourselves and is what is real for us. We live by these ideas and emotions and they give rise to our actions. Even if our perceptions are distorted and erroneous, they direct our behaviour, and, as we are the people who know ourselves best and can take responsibility for ourselves, we are best qualified to know what directions to take to grow and change. Rogers observed that the perceived 'self' influences our behaviour quite radically. For example, if I view myself to be competent and confident, I perceive and act within the world very differently from how I would if I experience myself to be incompetent and anxious.

According to Rogers, we evaluate every experience in relation to our self-concept and are motivated to behave in a way which is consistent with our self-image. If experiences are consistent with our knowledge of ourselves, we can incorporate them with ease and continue to hold the same self-concepts. In other words, the experiences of the organism are in harmony with the self-concept; they are 'congruent' and both influence behaviour. However, many experiences we have are not consistent with our self-concepts and may be threatening to the view we hold of ourselves. If that be so, Freudian type defence mechanisms may operate. We can deny our experience, a process I will look at later, or accept the experience and adjust the self-concept to accommodate it. The following illustrates these ideas. I have a view of myself as a good driver and I am always attentive to what I am doing whether on the motorway or country lane. I have an accident. I misperceive the speed of another vehicle and hit another car. This certainly does not fit in with my self-concept and I am very upset about the event. I may find the experience so painful and threatening to my self-concept, that I deny (and this can be at an unconscious level) any responsibility for it, and blame the other driver through projection, even though it is apparent to observers that such is not the case. Or, I can take responsibility, recognise the part I played in the event and adjust my concept of myself from one of being a good driver to one which acknowledges that I am not always as good as I would like to be. The more experiences are denied because they are not consistent with our self-concept, the greater the divide between self and reality. Indeed we become 'incongruent' and must defend ourselves from the reality of experience, for it is too painful to accept the truth. As more and more experiences are denied awareness, the self loses touch with reality and we become more and more maladjusted. Because we do not trust our sense of being, we live according to preconceived plans rather than living existentially.

The interpretation of experience in relation to self-concept also makes it difficult for us to fully understand each other. I can only understand you and your actions as I experience and interpret them according to my values, beliefs and attitudes. I cannot interpret them in the light of your experience, values, attitudes and beliefs for they are probably unknown to me. Consequently I may not understand you at all, although I may claim to. You will recognise in the acceptance of the subjective reality the phenomenological perspective of Rogers' position.

Ideal self

Not only is the self-concept important in Rogerian theory but so is the 'ideal self'. He found that we seem to carry within us an idea of what we would ideally like to be. We have some recognition of who we are and can describe ourselves to some degree, but we also have a concept of who we might be. The difference between the self-concept and the ideal self influences behaviour, for if there is a large gap between the two, and the ideal is unattainable, the individual will strive to achieve the ideal, but fail, for it is too unrealistic. The greater congruence (closeness and harmony) between the self-concept and the ideal the greater the happiness and sense of fulfilment.

Psychopathology

Like plants, each of us grows well if nurtured in a suitable environment. For human beings it is an environment of love, trust, acceptance and respect from significant others. It is Rogers' belief that the development of the well-adjusted person depends upon the individual receiving 'unconditional positive regard'. By that he means that each one of us needs to be accepted for who we are, and nurtured in an environment of love, warmth and trust. A child is the recipient of such love when she runs in from school waving a picture she has drawn that day, puts it under her mother's nose saying, 'Look what we did at school today, Mummy'. Her mother looks, smiles and approves by saying, 'Well done, it is lovely'. Approval is given and the child builds into her own self-concept approval for her activities and her sense of achievement and thereby, being. If, however, her mother is concentrating on something else and pushes the child aside abruptly because she cannot bear to be interrupted, the rejection and lack of approval will impede the child's development and her sense of worth. Approval or lack of it are very powerful forces that influence the child's growth and development, particularly that of the self-concept.

Rogers argues that being loved and accepted is a basic human need if we are to grow into fully functioning adults. He found that, in the course of growing up, children frequently experience a withdrawal of positive regard by parents when they have done something 'wrong'. I have heard such messages myself in Woolworths: 'Shut up; Mummy won't love you if you don't behave'. Good behaviour elicits love and acceptance, i.e. positive regard; bad behaviour results in threats of no love. The messages to the children are that only certain types of behaviour, those which parents label as 'good', are acceptable and will elicit love, and we leave children to find out what they are. It is a small step for children to move from 'some of my behaviour is not acceptable' to 'I am not acceptable'. All children have a strong curiosity drive and explore their world, and when parents apply conditions to the expression of their love, children hear and begin to believe that they are of little value and not worthy. Because all children need and wish to have love, they strive harder to gain it by behaving in a way that is acceptable to others, rather than in a way that enhances 'the self'. Stress and conflict may ensue. It is possible for us to be so anxious to please others in order to be accepted, that we lose touch with knowing our real selves.

In the well-adjusted person, both the 'self' and the 'organism' are working in harmony initiating and controlling behaviour, with the result that there is consistency between the self and the experience of the organism. The experience we have of an incident or event and our response to it fits in with our self-concepts—the persons we believe ourselves to be. There is no conflict, no disharmony; congruence prevails. On the other hand, if the experience does not fit in with the concept that one has of oneself, a discrepancy exists; then the person is in a state of 'incongruence'. I have a friend who, I believe, sees himself as an attractive, helpful, interesting and gentle person. He insists in telling me about his past adventures and trips abroad, the exotic places he has visited and the important people he has met. His speech is slow, ponderous, rather pompous and full of 'I'. I am sure my perception of him (and that of my friends for I have checked), that he is a bore, bears no relation to his own self-concept. If he observed me closely when talking, he would see the signals of tedium I emit—expressing a wish that he would get on with it—but his perception is distorted. The messages I give say one thing, but he sees another. The discrepancy between his experience of me and his self-concept would be painful to acknowledge and so reality is denied perception. Robert Burns wrote, 'O wad some Pow'r the giftie gie us to see oursels as others see us!'. If we do become aware of inconsistencies we can then change our behaviour or, as said before, accept ourselves as we are which may mean modifying our self-concepts and becoming more in touch with reality.

Application

Rogers accepted Freud's view that the defence mechanisms operated to protect the self from pain and distress. We need them at times to live comfortably, but excessive use can impede our growth and limit our development as full beings. Occupational therapists may well find that they are working with people who, for some reason, deny the awareness of their experience of events because they are too painful to handle. Excessive use of defence mechanisms results in 'neurotic' behaviour, because our actual behaviour is too far out of step with our concepts of self. As we deny the awareness of more and more experiences, we lose touch with reality and become more vulnerable to anxiety and more and more maladjusted. The loss of contact and knowledge of self each person experiences is accompanied by a lack of ability to live existentially and genuinely, for we can no longer trust ourselves. We no longer have a feeling of being in control and of having freedom of choice and therefore plan and live according to preconceived ideas, feeling manipulated rather than living openly to every experience. The tension created by living in this state may interfere in a person's life to such a degree that the whole personality becomes damaged.

Requirements for change

For human beings to embark upon the reintegrative process and become 'fully-functioning' again, we must lower the conditions of worth we have placed upon ourselves and thereby reduce our internal incongruences. This is not easy and only likely to occur if we receive unconditional positive regard from other significant people in our lives. We need to feel accepted just as we are, irrespective of our values, beliefs and behaviours. Unconditional acceptance by others promotes development and a growth of personhood as we reduce our defensive behaviour and open ourselves to new experiences which express and enhance our being. This is the basis of the person-centred therapy of Rogers. However, such does not happen in a vacuum. Rogers observed that one particular type of relationship more than any other was influential in promoting change. Truax & Carkhuff (1967) investigated his observation and found that the characteristics which facilitated growth are genuineness (sincerity), warmth and empathy and the ability to appreciate another person's point of view from his or her standpoint. Empathy means entering another person's private perceptual world, being sensitive to what is going on in that person and responding to that without making judgements. It is only possible for us to do this if we are comfortable and secure in our own perceptual world, knowing that we will not get lost in the other person's world, which will be different from our own and may even appear bizarre. We do this when we listen and try to understand our friends without criticism. We may show sympathy, but in our busy judgemental society empathetic listening is very rare and requires great skill.

Group work

This is of particular interest to me as much of my own teaching in the past has been person-centred work in groups. A group provides the opportunity to relate to many different people and we can learn so much about ourselves as we interact with others who have different phenomenal perspectives; the richness of the processes which arise between people cannot be measured.

In the late 1960s and the 1970s, Rogers became more involved in the use of groups as a medium of change and recorded his views on the place of encounter groups in human growth in 1970. Working in groups extends the application of the principles of humanistic psychology and enables us to meet others in a warm, supportive atmosphere where we can develop trust and confidence. In such a climate we can take risks, let down our defences, remove our masks, and stop striving to be something that others want us to be rather than being ourselves. We may get in touch with those aspects of our being which we thought others would not like, such as our anger or despair, and explore the reality of them for ourselves in a genuine way. We do not have to be what others want us to be and deny part of our being in order to be accepted; there are no conditions of worth. We may tentatively reintegrate painful experiences and may become more spontaneous in the expression of feelings. We receive from others their positive experiences of us in truth and trust. Sometimes this may be easy to accept, for the words are in accord with what deep down we know of ourselves, but at others it may lead to confrontations. Then we may feel vulnerable, and confrontations need gentle and sensitive handling by all members of the group, not just the facilitator. When we realise that whatever we say in truth is acceptable and that others strive to understand us, we are able to integrate parts of our own experiences, we are taking the first steps in the process of growth.

The qualities of the relationships within this type of group are parallel to those which we as occupational therapists need to establish in any group with which we work, if we wish to be agents of change. It does not matter if it is a practical activity group or a creative therapies group, the characteristics required for change are warmth, genuineness, empathy and unconditional positive regard. As a method of treatment this will be discussed later in Chapter 9.

Summary

From the outlines of the main tenets of the theories of Maslow and Rogers you will realise that they differ in many ways, but do have a great deal in common. In general, humanistic psychologists have a belief in the goodness of human nature and that people have an innate drive to grow, create and love. We have the power to make choices through which we may direct our own lives. Healthy growth and development depends upon the environment providing us with the necessary prerequisites. The fully mature person will then be more open, congruent, accepting and develop his or her full genetic potential. Without the right environment, we may grow up stunted, become aggressive and defensive, and maladjusted behaviour will ensue. The acceptance of our own experiences as valid evidence of our functioning makes research in the humanistic tradition difficult but not impossible. Maslow discusses the methods of research appropriate for this approach and more can be found in Reason & Rowan (1981) and Fransella (1982). Thus perspective keeps the person as a whole entity at the centre of study, even where there is illness or psychological disturbance. Such processes are not considered in isolation from the person. As such it rightly earned the title 'a person-centred approach' and has a valuable contribution to make to the practice of occupational therapy.

THE CURRENT STATE OF HUMANISTIC PSYCHOLOGY IN BRITAIN

In the three decades of the 1960s, 1970s and 1980s, humanistic psychology spread from the United States of America to Britain and then across Europe to Asia. Person-centred thinking extends beyond the bounds of psychology, counselling and psychotherapy to the thinking and practice of other disciplines where it challenges many of the well-established attitudes of work, politics, economics and social issues. It is only possible to cover a few aspects of the expansion in this field, so in the main the ones mentioned are those with which I am familiar.

Perhaps the recognisable face of humanistic psychology can be said to have appeared in Britain in 1969, for two major events occurred in that year. Firstly, a group of interested people met together and launched the Association of Humanistic Psychology (AHP) in this country and, secondly, Quaesitor (meaning seeker) the first centre for personal growth was established. The people involved were very active in promoting humanistic psychology and disseminated their ideas and thinking through the *Journal of the Association of Humanistic Psychology* which started publication in 1971. *Self and Society* appeared 2 years later and subsequently became the *European Journal of Humanistic Psychology*. In 1972, some members ran seminars for a wider academic audience at the annual conference of the British Psychological Society. Humanistic psychology had become a part of the acceptable national psychological scene.

The Psychology and Psychotherapy Association, a multidisciplinary organisation, came into being in 1973, and states its goals to be: to explore the implications of making the person central to psychological enquiry, psychotherapeutic practice and teaching. The Association runs workshops and training meetings and publishes *Changes* as an international journal. The British Association of Counselling grew rapidly and many members work within the person-centred philosophy. Both organisations are open to people from a variety of backgrounds (teachers, nurses, priests, occupational therapists) for whom a person-centred approach is a tenet of their work. Training opportunities grew yearly and in 1980 five proponents of Rogerian person-centred philosophy ran the first workshop of the annual Facilitator Development Institute (FDI) in Britain. The stated purpose of FDI is to help people become more effective with others. The main event is the annual workshop run in the summer as an intensive 8-day group experience where one can increase self-awareness and learn about one's capacity for growth and development in a climate of trust and mutual respect. My experience at FDI workshops enabled me to learn a great deal about myself, particularly in relation to personal responsibility and relationships with others.

Entry into the world of education came through a number of formal ways as well as informal. The MA in humanistic psychology at the University of Antioch was created in 1977 and the Institute for the Development of Human Potential at the University of Surrey was established in 1978. The University of Nottingham established an MEd in Human Relations, an experiential course which comprised personal growth as part of its syllabus, whilst institutes of higher education established training courses for counsellors within the humanistic psychological framework. In spite of some opposition, an art therapy course grounded in Rogerian theory was established by Liesl Silverstone in, and later validated by, Crawley College. Participants explained their own activities and creations to gain insights and growth without reliance on psychoanalytical assumptions and interpretations (Silverstone 1993).

Medicine has not escaped the influence of the phenomenological approach, although the route travelled by ideas may not be the same as for other disciplines. 1983 was the year that some members of the British Medical Association, being aware of the limitations of the biomedical model of disease, launched the British Holistic Medical Association. People are viewed as whole beings, who struggle to understand their place in the world and maintain health in daily life. The holistic approach in medicine assumes that all patients can take greater responsibility for their own health; consequently the emphasis is on education and negotiation rather than on physician determined treatment. Patrick Pietroni presented a guide to self-care with the title *Holistic Living* in 1986.

If people are to be studied as whole organisms, the logical positivist approach of experiment and laboratory work is antithetical to the humanistic philosophy and is not appropriate as a basis of study. In an attempt to redress the balance in the methodology of research, a group of members of AHP worked together and, in 1981, under the editorship of John Rowan and

Peter Reason, produced *Human Inquiry; a Sourcebook of New Paradigm Research*. Since that publication, a number of texts have been published stressing the need to adopt different approaches to the study of the person and I am delighted to find Colin Robson's (1993) publication, *Real World Research*, which puts the person at the centre of investigation.

The spreading of humanistic psychological ideas through associations, journals and events was accompanied by a growth in literature. The most comprehensive compendium being *Ordinary Ecstasy* (1976) by John Rowan, thoroughly revised in 1988. Writers such as Dorothy Rowe, David Smail, Brian Thorne, Ernesto Spinelli and Robert Ornstein all work within, or draw on ideas encompassed by, the humanistic perspective of human beings. For many people there is a desperate yearning for a psychology that leads to an understanding of the person as whole being, a member of the human species in one world. Even so, the expansion of the 1970s and 1980s seems to have declined over the last few years. Society has changed and become both more materialistic and individualistic. We are exhorted to strive to get on, make our own way in the world, to acquire material goods, and put on a good show. We are encouraged, (and our educational system is being reorganised to promote it) to acquire information, so that we can exercise knowledge and have skills to a level of measurable competency to compare ourselves with others. Is that what life is about? How can I know and be myself, be real, if I have to be something other than I am in order to put on a show? How do I develop my potential if the level of expectation is one of competency? Politics in humanistic psychology is about a way of living which accepts our attitudes and feelings for each other. It questions how men and women, straights and gays, adults and children, able-bodied and disabled, black and white, management and workers, even the Church and State relate to each other in this society. There are so many sections and segments in society for whom being in this world is riddled with misunderstandings and conflict. It was the knowledge of these divisions that compelled Carl Rogers, in his later years, to become involved in the processes of healing cultural divisions across the world, working for peace.

Many critics say the humanistic psychology is too idealistic. It does not deal with the realities of life. Others respond that it is because human beings are but children and have not yet fully developed that we find the ideas comprising humanistic psychology difficult to live by. The humanistic view is positive and constructive. It states that within the human organism the self is all right. It holds that when people are able to reduce defensiveness of the 'self' and become more open and responsive to social and environmental demands, reactions will be trustworthy and will enhance the organism. People do grow and change, they increase their experiencing and integration. It is an inherent process which is more than just daily living, for it encompasses creativity, spirituality and transpersonal experience.

CONCLUSION

From the evidence in this chapter, it is clear that the ideas of humanistic psychology with the emphasis upon the whole person, subjective experience and capacity for personal responsibility have made a valuable contribution to the understanding of human nature. Human beings are such complicated creatures that no one theoretical approach can encompass the whole truth about the species, but this specific school of thought contains fundamental differences from the behavioural and psychoanalytical approaches. The ideas of humanistic psychology have travelled a long way and penetrated many fields of work, particularly those concerned with human service. At one time Rogers referred to 'the quiet revolution' that was taking place as the influence of humanistic concepts spread to so many disciplines. In general, humanistic psychologists have a great belief in the goodness of human nature. They believe that human beings have an innate drive for growth, creativity and love, concomitant to a power to make choices through which they direct their own lives. Healthy growth and the development of the full genetic potential depends upon the features for growth being available within the environment. Just like plants, without the right environment, growth can be stunted. If we are unable to meet our basic needs, and loose touch with aspects of our being, we may become defensive or aggressive to a degree where we can adopt inappropriate, maladjusted behaviour.

It has to be noted that the greatest growth of humanistic ideas, and the hope that they promote, coincided with a period of economic expansion as the world became smaller through technological advancements and distant peoples became neighbours. The late 1980s and the 1990s have seen a change. World recession has occurred and, with it, what seems to me the development of a paradox. At the same time as individualism has come to dominate our lives wherein we must all take greater responsibility for ourselves in work, health, insurance and pensions for the future, the conditions which enable us to develop our potential and therefore take advantage of 'getting on our bikes' are becoming limited to a smaller section of our society. Humanistic psychology, like social psychology, believes that human behaviour is a function of both the person and the situation. If the situations are not those which encourage growth, human beings are diminished thereby.

As humanistic psychology places the person as a total entity at the centre of study, even where there is illness and psychological dysfunction, it rightly earns the title 'person-centred' and is a most appropriate theoretical framework for occupational therapists.

REFERENCES

Burns R B 1979 The self concept. Theory, measurement, development and behaviour. Longmans, London
Fransella F 1982 Psychololgy for occupational therapists. British Psychological Association/Macmillan Press, London
Maslow A H 1968 Towards a psychology of being. D Van Nostrand, New York
Maslow A H 1970 Motivation and personality, 2nd edn,. Harper & Row, New York
Mearns D, Thorne B 1988 Person centred counselling in action. Sage Publications, London
Nelson-Jones R 1982 The theory and practice of counselling psychology. Holt Rinehart & Winston, London, p 18
Ornstein R E 1975 The psychology of consciousness. Penguin Books, Harmondsworth
Person-Centred Review 1990 Special issue. Fiftieth anniversary of the person-centred approach. Person-Centred Review 5(4)
Pietroni P 1986 Holistic living: a guide to self care. J M Dent, London
Reason P, Rowan J (eds) 1981 Human inquiry: a sourcebook of new paradigm research. Wiley, Chichester
Robson C 1993 Real world research. Blackwell, Oxford
Rogers C R 1951 Client centered therapy. Constable, London
Rogers C R 1959 A theory of therapy, personality and interpersonal relationships, as developed in the client-centred framework. In: Koch S (ed) Psychology: a study of science, (Study 1, Vol 13). McGraw Hill, New York
Rogers C R 1969 Freedom to learn. Charles E Merrill, Ohio
Rogers C R 1970 Encounter groups. Penguin Books, Harmondsworth
Rogers C R 1975 Empathic: an unappreciated way of being. The Counselling Psychologist 3(2): 2–10
Rogers C R 1980 A Way of being. Houghton Mifflin, Boston
Rogers C R 1983 Freedom to learn for the 80's. Charles E Merrill, Ohio
Rogers C R 1990 (Edited by Kirschenbaum H and Henderson V L) The Carl Rogers reader. Constable, London

Rowan J 1983 The reality game: a guide to humanistic counselling and therapy. Routledge & Kegan Paul, London
Rowan J 1988 Ordinary ecstasy. Humanistic psychology in action, 2nd edn. Routledge, London
Rowan J 1990 Subpersonalities. The people inside us. Routledge, London
Shaffer J B P 1978 Humanistic psychology. Prentice Hall, New Jersey
Silverstone L 1993 Art therapy—the person centred way. Autonomy Books, London
Spinelli E 1989 The interpreted world: an introduction to phenomenological psychology. Sage Publications, London
Truax C B, Carkhuff R R 1967 Towards effective counselling in psychotherapy: training and practice. Aldine, Chicago

Cognitive change

Moya Willson

INTRODUCTION

Theories related to learning have always had a major influence on the practice of occupational therapy. Classical and operant conditioning underlie a number of techniques that are used to bring about changes in observable behaviour. Whilst often not observable, except indirectly through the spoken word, 'thinking' can be regarded as a form of behaviour. In this sense, a fixed set of ideas about ourselves and our environment can become a factor in our own anxiety, unhappiness and inadequate strategies for coping.

This chapter is about errors in thinking and the way in which 'cognitive therapists' perceive such problems and their solutions. The methods which they use owe a great deal to the usual procedures of behaviour modification. However, the terminology, and acknowledgement that the person is himself capable of being the creative force within his own change and development, reveals a humanistic orientation. All therapies are an attempt to create a satisfactory experience of living out of an essentially untidy world. The essential prerequisite to making sense of this material is to have a good working knowledge of both behaviouralism and humanism. It would also be useful to recognise that the work of certain theorists of personality development forms another cornerstone. Kelly's 'Personal Construct Theory', for example, makes useful background noises when considering Beck's approaches to cognitive therapy.

The first idea to consider is that your way of thinking about yourself and about what is happening forms the major contribution to how you feel. The second is that thinking is simply a form of behaviour which can be learned, unlearned or replaced like any other activity. In short, you are what you think but you can change your mind.

COGNITIVE RESTRUCTURING
Conceptions and misconceptions

The prevailing pattern of attitudes, beliefs, concepts, attributions or assumptions can be referred to as an individual's cognitive 'structures'. These form a basis for reasoning, for interpreting the present and for predicting the future.

Look at the pattern of nine dots in Figure 5.1.

Now take a pencil and, without lifting the point from the paper, join up all the dots using four straight lines. Spend a few minutes on this puzzle if you need to.

If this proved difficult, or if you still cannot do it, you have probably been thinking within the confines of an assumed square. This 'structure' has prevented you from solving the problem. Extend the pencil lines beyond the imaginary boundaries of this square and the problem can be tackled more effectively (see Fig. 5.3, p. 109).

This is a highly simplified example of how a self-imposed cognitive structure which is inaccurate or limiting can defeat our attempts to solve a problem or to complete a task. On a different level I may hold opinions about myself which lead me to avoid certain social events or practical tasks with which I believe myself unable to cope. The way in which we interpret the world and the beliefs we hold are not, however, always negative or

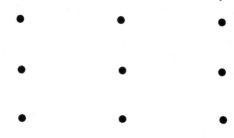

Figure 5.1 Nine dots.

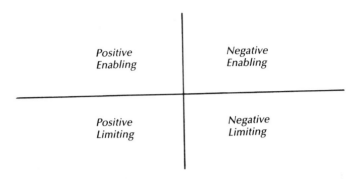

Positive Enabling	*Negative Enabling*
Positive Limiting	*Negative Limiting*

Figure 5.2 Positive/negative and enabling/limiting.

limiting. They may be positive and enabling. Try to generate some ideas about yourself which fit into the categories given in Figure 5.2.

If you have some difficulty in the 'negative enabling' box, then perhaps you never do anything which is deceitful, illegal or cruel.

The important thing to determine is the validity of the structures which direct our behaviour and emotional responses. For this reason, although every theorist in the field seems to use different descriptive terminology, Raimy's choice of the words 'conceptions' and 'misconceptions' seems particularly apt.

Conceptions are the psychological tools we use to organise and deal with not only the world around us but also our thoughts and feelings. Faulty conceptions, however, are likely to defeat us in both the external and internal worlds because they are erroneous maps or guides.

Raimy 1985

Of the many misconceptions we may have, leading to a variety of social and practical difficulties, he goes on to comment that:

Misconceptions about the self, however, are the most likely to produce defeat, disruption, maladjustment and neurosis. These misconceptions become anchored in the self concept, where as faulty guides to dealing with ourselves they often create havoc. Faulty beliefs about the self are particularly malignant because we always act upon them since they are the only guides we have to ourselves.

Identifying misconceptions

If we accept that misconceptions (or logical errors, false assumptions or irrational beliefs) are responsible for maladaptive behaviour or emotional disorders, then these misconceptions become the target of therapy. It therefore becomes necessary to identify them as closely as possible. The major clues are how the client feels and what he says both about himself and to himself. To try to separate feelings from thoughts or statements is, of course, rather artificial. As Lazarus (1972) comments: 'Cognition and emotion are usually fused in nature', and there is general agreement that emotions, as perceptual processes, are bound to have some cognitive content.

Bear in mind that it is not what happens which disturbs or upsets us but the way we see what is happening. Lazarus suggests that the important process is one of *appraisal*. We first appraise the relevance and potential benefits or threats of any situation. Then we appraise how we can cope with the situation in order to derive protection or advantage; after that we re-appraise the situation and our handling of it for future reference. In this way, our emotions can be understood in terms of an appraisal which mediates between a situation and our experience of it. Think about being anxious about an examination or excited about meeting someone and this should begin to make sense. Schachter & Singer (1962) pursue this line a little further showing emotion to be dependent not only on a physiological state of arousal but also on the way a subject *labels* or interprets this state. The way you label your emotional experience is in turn dependent on what you believe to be its origins. Here again we can make mistakes. We can misinterpret our own emotions or what has caused them or enter a situation with expectations (true or false) which mediate our behaviour and our emotional response. This is perhaps why it is easy to think oneself hurt when in reality the emotion is anger. Meichenbaum (1976) summarises work in this area by commenting 'how one responds to stress in large part is influenced by how he appraises the stressor, to what he attributes the arousal he feels, and how he assesses his ability to cope'.

Describing your own emotions or opinions *about* yourself and your capabilities is a way of talking about yourself, even if the words are not spoken out loud. The other component of self-verbalisation is talking *to* yourself, and this also can influence your emotional state. You talk *to* yourself about the prevailing situation, about what you are doing and about the likely outcome. To illustrate this whole area of self-statements and verbalisations, imagine the following scenario. You are baby-sitting in a friend's house and their Alsatian dog unexpectedly goes into labour.

Headings of different types of verbalising are given in Box 5.1; add your own likely responses.

Box 5.1 Theory into reality

Opinions about self
1. I can probably cope with this. I usually manage somehow.
2. I don't know what to do. I panic in situations like this.
3. I'm clumsy, and I don't like dogs anyway.
4.
5.
6.

Perceptions of the situation
1. It's a natural phenomenon, so she'll probably cope.
2. They should have told me this might happen.
3. This is an appalling crisis.
4.
5.
6.

Self-instruction
1. Keep calm; talk to her quietly.
2. Wait a minute, and it will be OK.
3. I'm feeling sick. I'm going to faint.
4.
5.
6.

Monitoring the situation
1. This is interesting. I'll be dining out on this one.
2. Something's bound to go wrong. They'll die.
3. I should have sent for help.
4.
5.
6.

It is easy to extract from such an exercise that some statements are positive and lead to an enhanced ability to solve problems and to cope. Conversely, the negative statements are more likely to lead to an experience of defeat and escalating anxiety. So why do people consistently use negative self-statements, thus decreasing their own ability to act effectively? Humanistic and behavioural psychology provide different but complementary answers—return to Chapter 4 for reasons relating to the development of self-concept. Behaviourally speaking, negative self-statements may often be positively reinforced by subsequent events. A situation arises which provokes an experience of mounting anxiety ('this is frightening'). Negative self-statements are generated ('I can't manage this. Other people do it better than me'). No risks are taken ('I'm useless, so there's no point'). Anxiety levels go down ('I have excused myself'). Someone else copes with the situation ('negative self-statements have saved me again'). When a difficult question is asked of a classroom full of students, how many of them use negative self-statements to reduce personal anxiety and to justify not attempting to answer it? The problem created by such a strategy is that positive reinforcement may be gained in the short-term, through reduction of threat-related anxiety, but there are long-term risks of damage to self-esteem and higher levels of anxiety due to lack of experience of success. Refer yourself to T. S. Eliot's poem 'The Love Song of J. Alfred Prufrock' while thinking about this. Prufrock does not provide a neat textbook example but contributes much more subtlety to this somewhat crude dissection of concepts.

In terms of therapy it is important to help the client to identify the negative self-statements that he uses within situations that he finds difficult or when his mood is disturbed or low. Once identified, their validity can be tested or positive alternatives sought. In the case of misconceptions to do with capability, Raimy warns us that clients may have, as well as real incapabilities, a confusion between being *unable* and being *unwilling*. When you say 'I can't tell my mother that I'm not going home for Christmas', do you mean that you lack the ability or that you choose to avoid the performance and its consequences? Many other statements which commence 'I can't think about', or 'I could never learn to' or 'I can't consider' may also fall into the category of things which one wishes to avoid irrespective of capability. They are a useful avoidance strategy and, as such, open to similar reinforcement through stress relief.

The next part of this chapter will briefly describe some of the strategies used by noted cognitive therapists. It is not intended as a guide to practice but to whet the appetite for further study.

RATIONAL EMOTIVE THERAPY
The premise

Albert Ellis (1962) suggests that positive human emotions, such as feelings of love or elation, are often associated with or result from internalised statements, stated in some form or variation of the phrase 'This is good for me!' and that negative human emotions, such as feelings of anger and depression, are associated with or result from sentences stated in some form or variation of the phrase 'This is bad for me!'. He also maintains that a person's emotional response to a situation reflects the label he has attached to the situation, for example dangerous or pleasurable, even when that label may be inaccurate.

In pursuing happiness, the essential human task according to Ellis, we are aided to achieve basic goals and purposes by rationality. Something which is irrational is something which prevents or defeats us. Two basic human tendencies underlie the theory of rational emotive therapy. First of all, humans tend towards irrationality, irrespective of teaching and experience; this amounts to a natural tendency to make ourselves disturbed. Fortunately, the second human feature is the potential to work towards change in the pursuit of happiness.

To any situation we bring two different types of cognition: beliefs and inferences. Beliefs relate to the personal significance of any event, are evaluative and have a strong influence on our emotional response. Inferences are ideas we have about likely outcomes and the meaning of our own and others' behaviour. Ellis (1962) suggested that there is a repertoire of irrational beliefs commonly held within our culture. These are as follows:

1. The idea that it is a dire necessity for an adult human being to be loved or approved by virtually every significant other person in his community.
2. The idea that one should be thoroughly competent, adequate, and achieving in all possible respects if one is to consider oneself worthwhile.
3. The idea that certain people are bad, wicked or villainous and that they should be severely blamed and punished for their villainy.
4. The idea that it is awful and catastrophic when things are not the way one would very much like them to be.
5. The idea that human unhappiness is externally caused and that people have little or no ability to control their sorrows and disturbances.
6. The idea that if something is or may be dangerous or fearsome one should be terribly concerned about it and should keep dwelling on the possibility of it occurring.
7. The idea that it is easier to avoid than to face certain life difficulties and self responsibilities.
8. The idea that one should be dependent on others and need someone stronger than oneself on whom to rely.
9. The idea that one's past history is an all-important determinant

of one's present behaviour and that because something once strongly affected one's life, it should indefinitely have a similar effect.

10. The idea that one should become quite upset over other people's problems and disturbances.

11. The idea that there is invariably a right, precise, and perfect solution to human problems and that it is catastrophic if this correct solution is not found.

Ellis 1962

These are quoted at length because it is worth reading them carefully and assessing for yourself the extent to which these beliefs are responsible for your own occasional distress or unhappiness. If you agree that they are, then do you also agree that they are irrational? To Ellis, they are irrational because they are not likely to be supported by one's environment and yet people use them to label situations, thus determining their own ineffective behaviour and emotional distress. They are also stated in absolute terms such as 'must', 'should' and 'ought' which, when in conflict with reality, lead to negative emotions and maladaptive behaviour. Rational beliefs are non-absolute and indicate desires, preferences and wishes. They may lead to emotions such as pleasure, disappointment or concern but these are appropriate and do not prevent one from establishing new goals.

It becomes clear that accepting all of the above premises as a basis for strategic therapy implies that the therapist and client will be working towards profound philosophical change in the way in which the latter construes the world and assumes meanings. Ellis describes the dynamic process involved: 'In Rational Emotive Therapy, the therapist or teacher shows people how to vigorously challenge, question and dispute their irrational beliefs. Thus they are shown how to ask themselves: Why is it awful that I failed? Who says I must succeed? Where is the evidence that I am a worthless person if I fail or get rejected?' Through such disputing of beliefs the client is able to develop different ways of thinking, which allow him some measure of failure whilst confirming his validity as a worthwhile person. Dryden (1984) acknowledges the difficulties of this and the nature of the required relationship between therapist and client: 'In helping clients achieve such profound change, effective rational-emotive therapists are unswerving in their unconditional acceptance of their clients. They realise that the achievement of profound philosophic change is an extraordinarily difficult task, and one which frequently involves many setbacks.'

Practice

Within this strategy of teaching or persuading the client to label situations more rationally, the therapist and client must share clear goals. A client who is open to and capable of profound change may work towards accepting himself unconditionally, refusing to rate anything as 'awful' and increasing his tolerance to frustration, in short working towards Ellis' concept of positive mental health. Others may be more suited to more limited goals related to changing their responses to certain specific situations or drawing less distorted inferences.

The style of the therapy is actively directive and structured but may draw on a number of different techniques when they seem appropriate. The following stages and variations may be employed, depending on the needs of the client.

Explanation. The basic rationale of rational emotive therapy is explained to the client, examples being given of how expectations may direct emotional responses, how self-statements are made and situations labelled.

The client is shown how certain assumptions or beliefs are irrational and how adhering to absolutes (such as 'should' and 'must') leads to distress and frustration.

Assessment. The focus is turned on the client's own problems with emphasis on his own self-statements and beliefs. He is encouraged to test the rationality of these and their present consequences in terms of emotional responses and behaviour.

Modification. The client is taught to identify and to challenge his own self-statements which will lead him to re-evaluate his existing beliefs. As progress is made, new positive self-statements arise from a more realistic appraisal of situations. This is a lengthy process and may involve 'imaginal presentation' whereby imaginary situations are worked through in order to discuss the rationality of likely beliefs, inferences and emotional responses. Behavioural rehearsal may be carried out in preparation for homework assignments. Putting learning into practice in real life and then discussing the experience can be an important part of facilitating change. The therapist may also use modelling, not to dictate the client's responses to his own problem situations, but to demonstrate how the therapist is able to use rational re-evaluation to minimise frustrations within his own life. The client may also be referred to self-help books written on rational emotive therapy lines, such as Ellis & Becker's *A Guide to Personal Happiness* (1982).

COGNITIVE APPROACHES
Beck's cognitive therapy

Aaron Beck (1967, 1976) concentrated his attention on the way in which depressed people see themselves and interpret events. He suggested that their primary problem is illogical reasoning leading to distorted conclusions about themselves and about their immediate environment. The types of errors in thinking which such people make are easy to understand, because we all make them from time to time, especially when making mountains out of molehills or when blaming ourselves for everything. Beck suggests that the depressive is subject to arbitrary influence, selective abstraction, overgeneralisation, and magnification/minimisation.

- Arbitrary influence is when you think you are a failed human being because no theatre tickets are available for Saturday—or any other example of drawing conclusions about yourself without adequate evidence.
- Selective abstraction is when the team you play for loses and you blame yourself entirely, irrespective of how the others played.
- Overgeneralisation is when a low mark for one assignment serves as proof that you are unintelligent and unworthy and unlikely to finish the course.
- Maximisation is blowing up minor setbacks into major catastrophes and minimisation is when you fail to give credit to your own achievements or positive qualities; both are errors in self-evaluation.

The therapeutic strategies which arise from identifying these errors in logic are directed towards rectifying the errors, so that the depressed person can arrive at more positive conclusions about himself. This often means re-examining the 'evidence' on which conclusions have been based. For example if the client complains that he always feels miserable or that nothing he attempts ever succeeds, then the first step will be to keep an accurate record of feelings or events. Such a record is likely to reveal that there are times when misery is not present and that some tasks do turn out all right. The overgeneralisation or misconception can then be re-examined in the light of this revised factual base. If the client reports difficulty in attempting to do anything due to the apparent immensity of any projected task and the prediction of failure, then the strategy may be to select a task and to break it down into small manageable steps, each of which allows the experience of success. These apparently simple and 'common-sense' strategies have an essential element in common; the therapist is helping the client to change his way of thinking by carrying out experiments with a changed hypothesis. Thus 'I never can, therefore I won't' becomes 'I sometimes can, therefore it's worth trying'. This form of 'collaborative empiricism' can be used to challenge the illogical self-judgements which have turned the client into his own victim.

Self-instruction

When mastering a new and complex task many people use self-instruction to aid concentration and efficiency and to decrease anxiety. The typical example is learning to drive a car when a monologue: 'Mirror...OK nothing coming...indicator... change down...watch that dog...etc.' is often used to monitor the task. As experience and confidence are gained, the process becomes 'unconscious', re-emerging only in times of stress. In a crisis, whether driving, rock climbing, searching for lost keys or administering first aid, a similar technique is often employed to keep the situation under control: 'OK...think clearly...first try this ...not good...now move that...'.

Some people appear to use 'self-instruction' more than others and it can be taught, as a coping strategy, to clients who have difficulty in coping with stressful situations. Meichenbaum et al (1974) described the use of self-instruction in the management of fear, anger and pain. The client is helped to become more aware of the inner language he is currently using and to develop more adaptive 'self-talk'. In relation to fear or anxiety, the strategy has to be developed to cover four major phases of a stressful event, anticipation, confrontation, during threat of being overwhelmed and after coping successfully.

Thought stopping (Wolpe 1969). This apparently very simple strategy is a good example of thinking being amenable to the same behavioural controls as simpler forms of human activity. It can be used to disrupt distressing ruminations or other obsessional trains of thought. On the first few occasions the client is invited to embark on his habitual unhealthy pattern of thinking, and once this has been established the therapist makes a sudden loud noise or shouts 'Stop'. This naturally disrupts the mental process. After the first few such demonstrations the client comes to expect his thoughts to be disrupted—which is disrupting in itself. He should also learn to take over the therapist's role of providing the cue to stop, and for this a more discreet signal can be used such as snapping a rubber band worn on the wrist.

RELEVANCE TO OCCUPATIONAL THERAPY

Many of the ideas expressed here are not new to the practice of occupational therapy with its tradition of practicality and problem solving. Creake (1990) confirms that 'occupational therapists are concerned with cognitive dysfunction when it interferes with the individuals capacity to perform tasks competently and to fulfil normal life roles'. It is against this background that she describes assertiveness training, time structuring and the building of leisure skills as ways of developing positive self-image.

An important concept to therapists is that of enabling people to achieve a sense of mastery. In the use of practical activities this often refers to the mastery of constructive, creative or domestic skills. Learning how one's thinking and reactions to situations can influence emotional function is a step in achieving mastery of oneself and one's environment.

There are a number of features of these approaches which are already used very positively by occupational therapists. The most obvious is Beck's strategy of breaking down tasks into easy steps, each of which ensures an experience of success. Less commonly used, in an overt way, is self-instructional training although this is referred to within Chapter 8, in the context of anxiety management.

The more formal adoption of cognitive–behavioural methods has advantages, particularly when working within a multi-disciplinary team, since strategies can have shared intentions and are open to discussion and evaluation. The use of related assessment

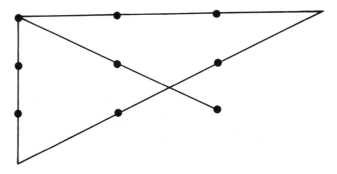

Figure 5.3 Nine dots joined by four straight lines.

measures, for example the 'Beck Depression Inventory' (Beck et al 1961) or the 'Dysfunctional Attitudes Scale' derived from Burns (1980), facilitate research into efficacy and treatment outcomes.

This chapter has focused on the principles upon which cognitive–behavioural approaches are based. It provides a structured, albeit confronting means, of bringing about personal change. The philosophy, however, leans more towards humanism than to its behavioural origins. Read in conjunction with Chapter 4 this becomes a powerful frame of reference within occupational therapy.

For those who came unstuck at the beginning of the chapter, Figure 5.3 gives the solution to the problem in Figure 5.1.

REFERENCES

Beck A T 1967 Depression: clinical, experimental and theoretical aspects. Harper & Row, New York

Beck A T 1976 Cognitive therapy and emotional disorders. International Universities Press, New York

Beck A T, Ward C H, Mendelson M, Mock J, Erbaugh J 1961 An inventory for measuring depression. Archive of General Psychiatry 4: 53–56

Burns D D 1980 Feeling good: the new mood therapy. Signet Nal Penguin, New York

Creake J 1990 Occupational therapy and mental health. Churchill Livingstone, Edinburgh

Dryden W 1984 Individual therapy in Britain. Harper & Row, New York

Eliot T S 1936 Collected poems 1909–1935. Faber, London

Ellis A 1962 Reason and emotion in psychotherapy. Lyle Stuart, New Jersey

Ellis A, Becker I 1982 A guide to personal happiness. Wilshire, North Hollywood

Lazarus R, Averill J 1972 Emotion and cognition with special reference to anxiety. In: Speilberger C (ed) 1972 Anxiety: current trends in theory and research. Academic Press, New York

Meichenbaum D H 1972 Cognitive modification of test anxious college students. Journal of Consulting and Clinical Psychology 39: 370–380

Meichenbaum D H 1976 Cognitive behaviour modification. In: Spence J, Carson R, Thibault J (eds) Behavioural approaches to therapy. General Learning Press, New Jersey

Meichenbaum D H, Goodman J 1971 Training impulsive children to talk to themselves. Journal of Abnormal Psychology 77: 115–126

Meichenbaum D H, Kanfer F H, Goldstein A P (eds) 1974 Helping people change. Pergamon Press, London

Raimy V 1985 Misconceptions and the cognitive therapists. In: Mahoney M J, Freeman A (eds) Cognition and psychotherapy. Plenum Press, New York

Schachter S, Singer J E 1962 Cognitive, social and physiological determinants of emotional state. Psychological Review 69: 379–399

Seigel L J, Peterson L 1985 Reducing stress in children's responses to repeated dental procedures. In: Mostofsky D I, Redmont R L (eds) Therapeutic practice in behavioural medicine. Jossey Bass, London

Wolpe J 1969 The practice of behaviour therapy. Pergamon Press, New York

6

Issues in community and primary care

Kim Atkinson

INTRODUCTION

With the continuing moves towards community care for people with mental health problems, occupational therapists in this field of practice are experiencing a shift in the framework in which they are working. In short-term psychiatry, hospital admissions are becoming shorter in duration and many people are treated solely within the community. There is an increasing demand for occupational therapists working in short-term psychiatry to be community based and to have more of a role within primary care teams. These wider changes have led to, and will continue to lead to, changes in the roles and working practices of occupational therapists working in short-term psychiatry.

This chapter addresses some of the issues relating to the practice of occupational therapy in short-term psychiatry in community and primary care. The client group will not be specifically defined, as the diversity within this field of practice is vast. It has been my experience that, when working in community care within short-term psychiatry, many of the clients have long-term needs. Issues particularly pertinent to work in short-term psychiatry are the focus of this chapter, but general issues for an occupational therapist working in community mental health are also addressed.

WHAT IS COMMUNITY AND PRIMARY CARE?

The concept of community care is vague and ill-defined (Bond & Bond 1986). Earlier definitions referred to the trend of replacing large and often geographically remote institutions with smaller residential establishments. The concept of community care now excludes care in most residential establishments of any size which are used on a permanent basis. It includes both health and social care provided by statutory, voluntary and independent agencies with a strong emphasis on personal and social networks (Compton & Ashwin 1992, Bond & Bond 1986). Community care involves providing services and support to enable individuals, wherever possible, to live as independently as possible within their own homes or elsewhere within the community (DoH 1990). In relation to short-term psychiatry this means that clients are more likely to receive care from community-based services rather than from services based in hospitals. It also means that wherever possible care will be provided in this way rather than through admission to hospital.

The momentum of community care has gradually increased since the concept was first mooted in the late 1950s and early 1960s (Health Service Journal 1993). At this time there was an emerging recognition that the most effective care may not be provided in institutional settings with their emphasis on control and custody (Goffman 1961, Murphy 1991). Since then, the progress of community care can be charted (Health Service Journal 1993) culminating in the most recent National Health Service and Community Care Act 1990.

Community care has been the subject of much controversy. There is some debate as to whether it means care in the community or care by the community. There has also been a disparity between the policy plans and what is actually happening in practice (Compton & Ashwin 1992, Warden 1993). While some community services are successful, others are often disorganised and fragmented. Successive governments have taken little interest in the provision of psychiatric services, and funding has been sporadic and often inadequate to implement the required changes (Murphy 1991).

Primary care is an integral part of community care. The concept of primary care has evolved since the start of the National Health Service (Davies & Davies 1993, DoH 1990). The role of primary health care is to care, to manage, educate about and prevent disease in physical, psychological and social aspects of life, in order to improve the quality of life (Compton & Ashwin 1992). Primary health care services are managed by district health authorities, general practitioners and primary health teams (DoH 1990). Either district health authority health centres or practice-owned surgeries are the focal points for the provision of primary care services. Delivery of efficient and effective primary care depends on close cooperation between various health professionals and occupational groups (Davies & Davies 1993). More recently, the primary health care team has developed and expanded to include practice nurses, therapy services including occupational therapy, health visitors, community psychiatric nurses and district nurses, for example (Compton & Ashwin 1992).

For occupational therapy, initially, much of the community practice of occupational therapists focused around providing services to people with physical disabilities. However, occupational therapists working in psychiatry recognised the need for a community occupational therapy service for their clients primarily with a focus on reducing readmission (Thomas 1987). The focus of community-based practice in psychiatry has considerably widened and occupational therapists are establishing their role within community and primary care services. Within this, their role focuses on preventing admission, facilitating early discharge and optimising independence. The occupational therapist in community and primary care in short-term psychiatry can, for example, be involved in activities of daily living and domestic rehabilitation work, social skills training, work training, relaxation therapy, counselling, carers' support, social and leisure activities and running support groups for clients (College of Occupational Therapists 1993, Sparling et al 1992).

POLICY FRAMEWORK

It is essential that occupational therapists working in short-term psychiatry in the community are aware of the framework of policies and legislation that they are working within. Occupational therapists working in the community are often working in relative isolation; decisions which the therapist previously took alongside a team with senior staff available now often have to be taken in relative isolation (Dimond 1988).

For an occupational therapist working in the community with clients with short-term mental health problems the most relevant legislation and policies include:

- the Mental Health Act 1983
- care management
- the care programme approach.

The Mental Health Act 1983

Sections 2, 3 and 4 of the Mental Health Act 1983 allow for compulsory admission of a client. Compulsory admission requires that there is evidence of a mental disorder and that the client needs to be detained in the interests of his or her own health and safety or for the protection of others.

- Section 2 allows for admission for assessment for up to 28 days.
- Section 3 allows for detention for treatment for up to 6 months; this may be renewed for a further 6 months and then for periods of 1 year. Detention should be necessary because essential treatment cannot be provided unless detained under Section 3.
- Section 4 is for use in emergency, requiring that compliance with the provisions of Section 2 would lead to an unacceptable delay. Section 4 allows for detention for up to 72 hours but does not allow for compulsory treatment (Dimond 1988).

Only the nearest relative or an approved social worker can apply for admission under any of these sections. It is very likely that at some point an occupational therapist working in short-term psychiatry in the community will have a client on her case-load who she believes requires detention under the Mental Health Act 1983. In practice, the nearest relative often initiates this procedure by telephoning a health professional they know the client has contact with. This may be the occupational therapist, particularly if she is the key worker, or it may be the general practitioner or community psychiatric nurse, for example. It is then the responsibility of that professional to ensure that the procedure is set in motion, usually in liaison with the consultant psychiatrist or the general practitioner. If the nearest relative does not initiate the procedure, and the occupational therapist is of the opinion that the client should be detained, the occupational therapist would need to contact the approved social worker, again usually in liaison with the general practitioner or psychiatrist.

The main provisions of the Mental Health Act 1983 that relate specifically to community care are the guardianship provisions. These are detailed in Section 8(1) of the Act and provide the power to require:

- the client to live in a specified place, and to attend specified places for medical treatment, occupation, education or training
- access to the client to be given to any registered practitioner, approved social worker or specified person.

At the time of writing, the most profound weakness is that there is no power to enforce the guardianship provisions and also no power to enforce a client living in the community to take any prescribed medication. These weaknesses have been acknowledged at policy maker level and new policies regarding these are likely to be introduced (Dimond 1988, Bluglass 1993).

Care management

The Government's plans for community care for the next decade and beyond are outlined in the White Paper 'Caring for People' and the National Health Service and Community Care Act 1990 (DoH 1990). Local authorities have the lead responsibility for community care (British Association of Occupational Therapists 1992) but they are to have very close links with health services, voluntary agencies, housing agencies and those in the independent sector (DoH 1990). One of the cornerstones of these policies is the implementation of care management, which came into full operation in April 1993.

It can be argued that care management has its strength in meeting the needs of people with long-term problems, through providing coordinated packages of care and having named, and thus accountable, key workers. However, it has a strong role within short-term psychiatry in helping to maintain a client within the community successfully, and the occupational therapist working in community-based short-term psychiatry should have an understanding of care management.

Care management ensures that:

- resources are targeted to where there is most need
- a comprehensive assessment of need is undertaken
- clients and carers are fully involved
- the service is flexible and speedy

- there is a clear plan and each profession or service is aware of its role
- value for money is maintained (Ovretveit 1992).

It involves three processes:

1. comprehensive assessment of need including the needs of the carer
2. design of a package of care agreed with the client, the carer and relevant agencies
3. implementation and monitoring (DoH 1990).

Through its systematic, documented and accountable approach, care management in community-based short-term psychiatry goes some way to ensuring that the needs of the vulnerable are met and that contact with the client is maintained and the appropriateness of services is monitored.

A number of different models of care management exist but generally, within the purchaser/provider concept introduced in the National Health Service and Community Care Act 1990, the care manager along with the client is the purchaser. The occupational therapist may find him- or herself in the role of care manager and thus a purchaser or he or she may be a provider of services (British Association of Occupational Therapists 1992).

Care programme approach

By April 1991, all health authorities were expected to have defined and implemented local care programme policies. These were to apply to all inpatients considered for discharge and new patients accepted by specialist psychiatric services (DoH 1990). The 1975 White Paper 'Better Services for the Mentally Ill' (DHSS 1975) set the framework in which care programmes would be introduced. This was endorsed in the 1989 White Paper 'Caring for People' (DoH 1989).

The care programme approach introduced a systematic arrangement for assessing whether a client could realistically be treated in the community within the given resources. It also ensured that proper arrangements were made for continued health and social care after discharge from hospital (DoH 1990). The exact form that the care programme approach takes varies locally and the use of care programmes is patchy (Groves 1993). Key workers are responsible for monitoring the plan and keeping in close contact with the client and other services involved in the care programme. Thus, contact with the client is maintained and the provision of services is monitored. In order to fulfil this responsibility, the key worker arranges regular reviews of the care programme to ensure that it is still meeting the client's needs. An occupational therapist may have the role of key worker for a client. Such a system helps to ensure that communication is maintained between the various services that are involved; this can be a difficulty in community care. Like care management, it also provides a measure to protect the needs of the vulnerable and maintain contact with clients in the community. Various arrangements are established at a local level to enable care management and the care programme approach to work together effectively and efficiently.

ISSUES FOR PRACTICE AS AN OCCUPATIONAL THERAPIST IN COMMUNITY MENTAL HEALTH

Role within the multidisciplinary team

In community mental health, the occupational therapist is likely to be working in closer contact with other members of the multidisciplinary team than in hospital-based psychiatry. The occupational therapist is unlikely to be working within a traditional occupational therapy department and will have a much closer working relationship with the multidisciplinary team, possibly being the only occupational therapist within that team.

Community teams have less structure than institutions (Feaver & Creek 1993). As such, the occupational therapist working within a community team has greater freedom to define and develop a model of practice and role. Working in professional isolation makes it important that occupational therapists are clear about what their role is. Along with other health professionals, occupational therapists are increasingly being placed in the position of having to justify their role and position; an integral part of such a process is a clear understanding of skills. Within a team, each professional has core skills, common skills and specialist skills (Joice & Coia 1989).

Core skills are essential for the effective completion of certain areas of work. It may be that other professionals can do certain elements of these skills, but only to a point. Each profession has its own core skills which reflect its particular expertise and elements which it places as a priority (Joice & Coia 1989). It is on this basis that multidisciplinary teams have their strength. There has been long-running debate within the occupational therapy profession about what our core skills are (Blom-Cooper 1989, Joice & Coia 1989, Thorner 1991, Westland 1985). Joice & Coia (1989) suggest that we have three core skills:

- the use of purposeful and meaningful selected activity
- activity analysis
- the assessment and treatment of functional abilities.

In relation to community-based practice in short-term psychiatry each of these core skills, and the philosophy in which occupational therapists work, are of relevance and value. The principles of community care which have been enshrined in the National Health Service and Community Care Act 1990 are about helping clients to achieve an optimal quality of life and independence. Within the philosophy of community care, this is to be achieved through promoting self-determination and autonomy in clients, involving them in the planning of their care and treatment, minimising segregation, creating as normal an environment as possible and using practical everyday solutions (Murphy 1991). The principles and philosophy of community care reflect the philosophy, role, core skills and working practices of occupational therapists who focus on the clients' context. In the selection of activities for treatment, the occupational therapist selects activities which are of relevance and interest to the client and the client's role within society. The activities are used to help the client achieve maximum independence and quality of life. Through activity analysis, the therapist can adapt an activity to the individual's environment or behaviour (Thorner 1991). Through the assessment and treatment of functional abilities, the therapist uses practical everyday solutions to promote independence and optimise quality of life.

As well as the core skills mentioned above, the occupational therapist also has common skills and specialist skills. Common skills are skills which are shared with other members of the multidisciplinary team. These may include skills such as counselling or group work (Joice & Coia 1989). Specialist skills are additional skills which any members of the multidisciplinary team may have acquired, usually through their own personal interest or opportunity, for example psychoanalytic therapy and aromatherapy (Joice & Coia 1989).

Isolation or autonomy?

Since community work lacks many of the structures which are in place in institutions such as hospitals, there are a number of issues surrounding isolation or autonomy to be addressed by an occupational therapist practising within the community. Some therapists will thrive on the autonomy of working in the community, on the lack of rigid structures and the opportunity to manage their own time. Others will feel isolated in such a position. The following section will discuss a number of issues about isolation and autonomy for the occupational therapist working in the community in short-term psychiatry.

Model of practice

The lack of structure which is evident in community practice also means that there is a less-dominant philosophy in place. In hospitals, the occupational therapist is usually constrained to working within the medical model, which does not fit comfortably with the philosophical base of occupational therapy. In the community, there is more opportunity for occupational therapists to practice according to their own professional philosophical base and within whichever model is most appropriate (Feaver & Creek 1993). This opportunity may not be capitalised on if, when working within a team, the team chooses a multidisciplinary approach. This leads to role blurring and the relinquishing of theoretical boundaries, leading to a pot of common skills but little recognition or use of the core skills of each profession within the team (Feaver & Creek 1993).

Supervision

An occupational therapist working in the community may be part of a multidisciplinary team where he or she is the only occupational therapist within the team. The occupational therapist may also be working in isolation from the rest of the team for a large proportion of the working week. These factors make the need for effective supervision important. Supervision should take the form of both clinical and professional supervision. Clinical supervision refers to supervision regarding the caseload; it may be appropriate to receive this from another occupational therapist or it may be provided by another member of the multidisciplinary team. Professional supervision refers to professional issues such as professional development and staff appraisal, for example. This would normally be provided by a more senior occupational therapist who may or may not be part of the same multidisciplinary team. The most important issue is that supervision is obtained from someone. Health care professionals often feel guilty at spending time in such a way and claim that they are too busy for such a luxury. The nature of community work in short-term psychiatry is very demanding, time for reflection is needed, and it is essential that workers receive the support and guidance that supervision provides if they are to be able to continue to offer a good quality service to clients (Compton & Ashwin 1992).

Clinical responsibility

When working in the community there is a considerable increase and broadening of responsibility. Decisions which were previously made as a team or in the support of a department are now often taken alone with the client in the client's home (Dimond 1988). At times, the community occupational therapist may be the only health professional in close contact with a client. He or she will need to make decisions regarding the client's mental state, which in a hospital setting could be discussed with medical and nursing staff who would be close at hand. If there is a deterioration in mental state, the community occupational therapist will need to decide at what stage this requires medical intervention or even at what stage sectioning procedures should be initiated. Occupational therapists in community-based psychiatric practice often find such a widening of clinical responsibility difficult to cope with. For this reason, junior staff are rarely employed in settings where they will be required to have such a clinical responsibility. More experienced staff in such a position will require support, close working relationships and good communication within the multidisciplinary team.

Time management

Community practice places the therapist in a more autonomous situation and in a situation where there are less structures in place than may be the case in hospital practice. To be able to work effectively and efficiently within such a setting requires developed time-management skills. Various time-management strategies may be adopted; a useful process in this is to obtain an accurate picture of how time is spent by monitoring working practices (Burnard 1992). This may help to identify how time-management skills may be improved and is something which could be discussed in supervision sessions.

Many community practitioners find it helpful to build structures into their working day. For example, they may choose to spend the first hour and the last hour of each day in the office. This provides a predetermined time to make and receive telephone calls, meet with other staff, deal with mail and write reports. Within community practice it is essential to build in structures which allow for free time. Free time is necessary in order to be flexible, to respond to the unexpected circumstances which often arise in community work. Working in community mental health is also demanding and stressful; free time provides an opportunity for reflection and helps to prevent the therapist from becoming overloaded. Because community work is so flexible it is very easy to lose free time.

Communication

When working in community mental health practice, awareness of the need for effective communication and the development of good communication skills are both of importance. A therapist working in such a setting may have little day-to-day contact with other members of the multidisciplinary team. In short-term psychiatry, situations can arise or change very quickly; these factors make communication within a team important.

As a staff group, communication helps to build team relationships, thus providing a support network for members of the immediate multidisciplinary team. Communication also helps the different team members to have a clear understanding of each other's roles and skills, which will lead to more effective working practices.

In community-based practice, communication goes beyond the multidisciplinary team. The nature of community work means that the therapist may be working with a whole range of community resources including health, social services and services within the voluntary or independent sector. The therapist may also be working very closely with the client's family or carers. Where more than one member of a team is involved with a client, communication between the various members is very important to ensure that the client is receiving the most effective intervention (Compton & Ashwin 1992).

Safety

There are certain issues related to safety that are likely to be more of a problem for the therapist working in a community mental health setting than for the therapist in a hospital setting. Most practices regarding safety are based on common sense but some teams may have specific policies and procedures in place which should be followed.

Because of the nature of some of the clients seen in short-term psychiatry, the therapist in community practice is likely to deal with some very disturbed clients in volatile situations. As a result of the mental illness the clients' perception may be distorted, they may be irritable and they are likely to feel confused and anxious. When working in the community, the therapist is in an exposed environment and on the client's territory'. Dealing with such a client requires some skill, and all therapists working in community psychiatry should consider safety precautions.

General practical precautions include:

- meeting clients for the first time at the health centre or clinic or with someone else present
- obtaining information from the referrer about risk factors
- informing others of the whereabouts of a home visit and expected return time—some teams have a book system in operation where such information is recorded
- asking another member of the team to become involved if worried or feeling insufficiently experienced.

Working process

The context of community work is very different from that of the hospital or similar institution. Many issues related to community work have been discussed. This section will focus on specific aspects of the day-to-day practice of an occupational therapist working in community-based short-term psychiatry.

Base

The first aspect is where the base of the community occupational therapist working in short-term psychiatry is likely to be. This varies from area to area; different teams and care groups are set up in different ways and some teams are more established than others. It is increasingly unlikely, however, that a community occupational therapist will be working within, or from, a traditional occupational therapy department.

Likely bases for an occupational therapist working in this field of practice include those of community mental health teams and general practitioner surgeries.

Commonly, occupational therapists working in short-term community psychiatry are based within community mental health teams. These teams normally consist of consultants, junior doctors, community psychiatric nurses and psychologists. Additional staff, such as a dietitian and specialists in alcohol or drug misuse, will have input. There will also be close working relationships with social services staff, in particular social workers and staff within the voluntary and independent sector. Such teams are usually based in a community-based facility such as a clinic or day hospital. Ideally, such a base will be geographically central within the area it covers and accessible to the community it serves, for example in the town centre or on a main bus route.

The community mental health team may work from the inpatient psychiatric facility. This may be the traditional psychiatric hospital or, increasingly, the psychiatry department of a district general hospital. Working from a hospital base has the advantage of enabling close liaison between the hospital and community services but it also maintains links with inpatient psychiatric care which some clients may find less acceptable.

As occupational therapy establishes its role within the primary care team (College of Occupational Therapists 1993) and as more general practitioners are moving towards being fund-holders, there is increasing demand for occupational therapists to be based within general practitioner surgeries. Within such a base, occupational therapists have been employed to work with clients with both physical and mental health problems and some have been employed to work within a particular specialism. Whether 'generic' or specialised, there is a role for therapists within this setting to work with people with short-term mental health problems (College of Occupational Therapists 1993, Sparling et al 1992, Westland, 1985).

Whether based in the community mental health team or in a general practitioner's surgery, the community occupational therapist working in short-term psychiatry may see clients at the base, in the client's home or in the wider community. Most community bases offer a number of interview rooms as well as treatment rooms with special facilities, for example a creative therapies workshop. Because of the nature of the practice of occupational therapy, much of the work of the occupational therapist will be carried out in the client's home or in the wider community. The occupational therapist may be involved, for example, in shopping with a client, participating in leisure activities or carrying out stress management programmes in the community setting.

There are a number of issues around the occupational therapy process—referral, assessment, intervention and evaluation along with recording and reporting of information—which are particularly pertinent to community practice in short-term psychiatry.

Referrals

When working in short-term psychiatry in the community, there are a number of issues related to referrals which are worthy of consideration. The first is that, when a therapist receives a referral for a client who is living in the community, the therapist has no clear knowledge of how well supported the client is. Such information is important when considering the priority of the referral.

The second issue is the source of the referral. When working in the community, referrals are likely to come from a variety of sources including self-referral. The referral is often the first knowledge the occupational therapist has of the client and, from this, the therapist draws cues regarding priority. When the referrer is known to the therapist, there may be better knowledge of the quality of the information provided in the referral; whether it will be detailed and accurate or vague and ill-defined (Grime 1990). When referrals come from such a wide range of sources in the community, the therapist does not always have this advantage.

The issues raised so far have been related to setting priorities and it may be useful to discuss, more specifically, how priorities are set in community-based short-term psychiatry. Some teams will have established priority standards which will have been agreed with the purchasers of their services. In most cases, priorities for clients seen in short-term psychiatry are based on the following factors:

- if the client has just been discharged from inpatient psychiatric care
- if there is a perceived suicide risk
- if the client has no support network or if this network has recently been altered.

On receiving a referral, the occupational therapist identifies specific cues within it that would place it as a priority. There is, however, always some uncertainty involved in such interpretation and the therapist should be aware of this (Grime 1990).

The issues of role blurring within the multidisciplinary team have already been discussed but they are also relevant here in relation to referrals. Multidisciplinary teams have different ways of allocating referrals to the various professional members. This process of referral allocation represents the perceived roles of the different team members. For this reason it is important that the occupational therapist receives referrals which require the core skills of occupational therapy as well as those referrals which draw on common skills and specialist skills.

Assessment

Occupational therapists regularly employ the assessment methods of interview, observation, standardised tests and self-rating scales (Finlay 1988). When working in the community, the same assessment methods are available to the occupational therapist but some additional considerations are relevant.

As a result of the National Health Service and Community Care Act 1990, a number of assessment batteries and schedules are completed with a client by a number of different agencies. Clients often find these demanding and intrusive and it may be appropriate for the occupational therapist to be sympathetic to this and make fuller use of other assessment methods. Most occupational therapists who work in community-based short-term psychiatry are experienced therapists with well-developed clinical reasoning skills. They are likely to feel easier about using observation and interview as their main assessment methods. In the less-structured environment of community care, standardised tests may not be so appropriate.

The final and most important point related to assessment is that, as a community practitioner, the occupational therapist has an opportunity to assess clients within their own context. Occupational therapy is about promoting independence within the client's environment and, with the opportunity to assess in this context, the assessment should be more realistic, accurate and meaningful.

Intervention

As well as assessments, the occupational therapist who is based in the community has opportunities to carry out interventions within the clients' own environment. This, however, raises some issues. Some clients may not wish to be treated in their home or local area and such wishes should be respected. As a community practitioner, the occupational therapist will often be a guest within the client's home and the client is at liberty to refuse any suggestions for treatment or alteration in lifestyle (Grime 1990).

When working with a client in the community, it is likely that others such as family members or the wider support network will be more involved. This may be more or less desirable and the implications of this should be recognised and considered with the client.

When working as community practitioners in short-term psychiatry, occupational therapist needs to be flexible in their working hours. In short-term psychiatry many of the clients are in full-time employment and therefore attending for treatment during normal working hours is not convenient. Mental health services are increasingly making themselves accessible in the evenings so that clients can receive treatment with minimal interruption to their employment.

Evaluation

Occupational therapists, along with all health professionals, are increasingly being asked to evaluate their work. In community-based practice, evaluation of occupational therapy intervention is particularly difficult. Measuring outcomes is difficult because much of the occupational therapist's role focuses on prevention and support. Within psychiatry, many other factors contribute to a client's mental state and ability to cope; for this reason it is difficult to attribute any outcome directly to the intervention of the occupational therapist. Quality issues are dealt with more thoroughly elsewhere in this book.

Recording information

The importance of effective communication as a community practitioner has already been discussed. An integral part of effective communication is recording information in written form. Other members of the multidisciplinary team may be involved with a client, and in short-term psychiatry circumstances can change quickly, making regular, accurate and succinct documentation essential. Because of the nature of community work, access to notes may be difficult; they may be kept in a central place and carrying clients' notes around in a car creates problems of security.

CONCLUSION

There are continued moves towards community care for people with short-term mental health problems. The concept of both community care and primary care has evolved over time. The principles and philosophy of community and primary care reflect the philosophy, role, core skills and working practices of occupational therapy and, as such, throughout their evolution occupational therapy has established a firm role.

The experience of working within the community is very different from that of hospital-based practice. Particular issues related to this have been discussed. The occupational therapist working in short-term psychiatry in the community works closely with the community care policy framework, fewer structures are evident and the therapist often works in professional isolation. Within the current climate, effective and efficient use of resources is essential and this has been discussed in relation to the importance of time management, supervision and effective practices in the occupational therapy process specifically relevant to community care.

REFERENCES

Blom-Cooper L 1989 Occupational therapy. An emerging profession in health care. Duckworth, London, p 43–56
Bluglass R 1993 Maintaining the treatment of mentally ill people in the community. British Medical Journal 306: 159–160

Bond J, Bond S 1986 Sociology and health care. An introduction for nurses and other health care professionals. Churchill Livingstone, United Kingdom, p 150-151, 156–157

British Association of Occupational Therapists 1992 National Health Service and Community Care Act, 1990: guidance for members. BAOT, London

Burnard P 1992 Effective communication skills for health professionals. Chapman & Hall, London, p 103–108

Compton A, Ashwin M 1992 Community care for health professionals. Butterworth-Heinemann, Oxford, p 7, 13, 257, 278

College of Occupational Therapists 1993 Occupational therapy in primary care. College of Occupational Therapists, London

Davies B M, Davies T 1993 Community health, preventative medicine and social services. Baillière Tindall, London, p 189–190

Department of Health 1989 White paper 'Caring for People'. HMSO, London

Department of Health 1990 Community care in the next decade and beyond. HMSO, London, p 3, 5, 23, 24, 75, 81

Department of Health and Social Security 1975 White paper 'Better Services for the Mentally Ill'. HMSO, London

Dimond B 1988 Mental health law and the occupational therapist. British Journal of Occupational Therapy 51(9): 307–311

Feaver S, Creek J 1993 Models for practice in occupational therapy. Part 2: What use are they? British Journal of Occupational Therapy 56(2): 59–62

Finlay L 1988 Occupational therapy practice in psychiatry. Chapman & Hall, London, p 37–53

Goffman E 1961 Asylums. Essays on the social situation of mental patients and other inmates. Penguin, England

Grime H 1990 Receiving referrals, decision making by the occupational therapist. British Journal of Occupational Therapy 53(2): 53–56

Groves T 1993 Closing mental hospitals. British Medical Journal 306: 471–472

Health Service Journal 1993 April is the cruellest month. Health Service Journal 103(5346): 11

Joice A, Coia D 1989 A discussion on the skills of the occupational therapist working within a multidisciplinary team. British Journal of Occupational Therapy 52(12): 466–468

Mental Health Act 1983 HMSO, London

Murphy E 1991 After the asylums. Faber & Faber, London, p 1–25, 42–59

National Health Service and Community Care Act 1990 HMSO, London

Ovretveit J 1992 Concepts of case management. British Journal of Occupational Therapy 55(6): 225–228

Sparling E, Clark N, Laidlaw J 1992 Assessment of the demands by general practitioners for a community psychiatric occupational therapy service. British Journal of Occupational Therapy 55(5): 193–196

Thomas C 1987 BJOT: occupational therapy in the community. British Journal of Occupational Therapy 50(10): 351–354

Thorner S 1991 The essential skills of an occupational therapist. British Journal of Occupational Therapy 54(6): 222–223

Warden J 1993 Politics of community care. British Medical Journal 306(6871): 166

Westland G 1985 Dipping into community mental health, an aspect of the occupational therapist's role. British Journal of Occupational Therapy 48(9): 260–262

7

Quality of care

Lynne Howard

INTRODUCTION

This chapter introduces the reader to the concept of quality of health care in short-term psychiatry. It examines what quality means to the therapist, manager and service user, by looking at the historical basis of quality measurement and suggesting a definition of quality for use in this setting. It explores the basic principles of quality assessment and the validity of various methods, looks at setting standards of care and the measurement of them and goes on to consider how these measures can contribute to good practice in occupational therapy.

Measuring quality in health care is not new. Sporadic efforts have been made over the years since Florence Nightingale's reports on levels of hospital-acquired infections during the Crimean War, but it was not until the late 1960s and early 1970s that quality issues began to be addressed in a systematic manner. In the UK, quality developments were driven by the need to ensure that expenditure on the NHS, in common with other public services, was producing value for money.

In the early 1980s, the move towards general management of the NHS and Sir Roy Griffiths' influential NHS management review (1983) injected the notion of consumerism into the service, and managers from industry entering the NHS brought with them some of the quality assurance initiatives and ideas of the business world. These fitted well with the Government's desire to promote competition and market forces in the service as a means of controlling costs and transferring power from the producers to the consumers of health care. However, many of the early initiatives were seen to be very superficial with little real choice for the consumer and of no challenge to the doctors' clinical freedom. Despite considerable interest, the measuring of effectiveness of treatments and processes of care within the NHS progressed little. Indeed, in 1988, the all-party Social Services Select Committee reported:

> The last major weakness of the NHS is that it is not possible to tell whether or not it works. There are no outcome measures to speak of other than that of crude numbers of patients treated. There is little monitoring on behalf of the public ... and the public and politicians cannot decide whether or not they are getting value for the resources pumped into the NHS.
>
> Social Services Committee 1988 (p. xi)

DEFINING QUALITY

Quality assurance initiatives have spawned considerable amounts of new jargon and a good deal of literature at all levels in the NHS. However, a concrete definition of quality in health care is hard to formulate. The British Standards Institute defines quality as 'the totality of features or characteristics of a product or service that bear on its ability to satisfy a given need' (BSI 1987). This echoes the requirements of manufacturing industry where consumer satisfaction is consistently demanded. Thus, the concepts of excellence and fitness for purpose are clearly part of defining quality. We have a customer, or consumer—the client—whose needs are to be met and a product—the action of the health care professional—which depends upon the needs that that action is intended to meet.

Thus consumer satisfaction is vital to a quality service, but Ovretveit (1990) suggests that the focus of the NHS in the mid-1980s was *either* on quality as providing customer satisfaction and choice *or* on professional standard setting and clinical audit. He suggests there is a danger in quality being equated with customer satisfaction alone, as may be the case in industry, because in health care the customers may not know what they need, perhaps requesting harmful or inappropriate treatment through lack of information, or not being in a position to exercise choice, as in the case of the very young or very severely incapacitated. Indeed, as Pfeffer (1992) suggests, most consumers have not chosen to be in need of health care and may find consumerism an additional burden. Thus, there is a place for professional definition of their needs.

The mid-1980s also saw attempts to measure the quality of health care with a managerial approach, using the quality control methods of industry. Williamson (1991) suggests that very little health service activity is capable of formal, industrial-type quality control. There, raw materials are purchased of known composition and predetermined quality. Standard procedures and processes are applied to them, the end products are inspected and substandard items are discarded. Health care is not so simple since other factors affect the outcomes of the health care process, such as the age, fitness and general health of the patient, other pathologies, the side effects of medication, unforeseen complications and much more. The patients are not standardised and the treatment regime is unique to the individual patient. Health care is not simply a matter of following protocols, but is judgementally based using training, past experience and expectation of outcome. In addition, the raw material is not inert—consumers have a view and can make judgements regarding the processes of care.

Bringing together the two strands of consumer opinion and staff definition of need we may formulate a definition of a quality service as:

> one which meets consumer needs (or fulfils their expectation of it) as perceived by them and by the staff who work within the service.

Thus, quality is not definable in a single measure but is a composite and, possibly, also a moving target, if there is to be continual improvement in a service. What is required of health care professionals is that they translate this abstraction into a process or activity which is graspable and achievable.

WHY MEASURE QUALITY?

For more than 30 years the Government has been concerned to promote quality in psychiatric care. 'The Hospital Plan for England and Wales' (DoH 1962) sought to put psychiatric units within district general hospitals, rather than isolate the patients in large out of town institutions. In 1975, the DHSS report 'Better Services for the Mentally Ill' reviewed progress towards more community management of psychiatric disorders, but found few non-hospital-based services in most areas.

More recently, the National Health Service and Community Care Act 1990 has split the NHS into purchasers and providers, with contracts between the two setting out what should be provided, to whom, at what cost, and with what quality guarantees. As the Department of Health guidelines state: 'the contractual process should be directed to improving the quality of services provided and not to efficiency and cost effectiveness alone' (DoH 1989).

The guidelines further require: 'The provision of systems to assure quality such as medical, nursing and other audits and surveys of patient opinion'.

Thus we have government-initiated requirements to measure service quality in addition to that which is done for the advancement of knowledge of techniques or settings which affect patients' functioning. There are also the quality initiatives carried out by the different professionals to measure their service inputs to the patients or clients. Most professionals would suggest that evaluation has always been integral to practice; the difference now is that it is to be formalised as comprehensively as possible and made known to those outside the professional group, such as members of the multidisciplinary team and managers.

A review of the literature reveals more research to have been published on monitoring and evaluating the quality of service provision to those in need of long-term inpatient care than has been done for patients with acute episodes or those in the community (Shepherd 1984, Lavender 1987, Perkins 1992). However, more work is now being carried out in these settings (Milne 1987, Dean et al 1993) and this will continue as our ability to measure quality in a wider range of settings improves.

The patient with mental health problems requiring an acute admission now remains in hospital for a much shorter time than would have been the case a few years ago. It might be tempting to imagine that the quality of care is not worth measuring over a relatively short period, but of course at any given time a patient is experiencing a certain quality of care and, whilst changes to the ward environment, for example, which takes place over a number of weeks, may not benefit that patient, changes will affect those who come after. Similarly, clients who spend a large proportion of their time in the day hospital have a right to a high-quality experience. The Patients' Charter (DoH 1991) encourages consumers to expect certain levels of service in health care settings. Shorter contact times with patients will influence the occupational therapy programme and we need to be able to show that our treatment methods are efficient, cost effective and of high quality if our services are to be purchased in the future.

A major difficulty of quality assessment is that it is not possible to directly attribute certain outcomes to antecedent processes of care. Many other factors impinge on our patients, and so we must do all we can to exert control over threats to the internal validity of any evaluation which may be carried out.

WHAT SHOULD WE MEASURE?

Thus far we have considered the background to quality measurement in the NHS, and reached a definition of service quality which can apply to the patient or client in short-term psychiatry. We have also explored why quality should be measured. The next step, therefore, is to ascertain what should be measured to arrive at an understanding of whether or not our service is of high quality. A framework is needed on which to hang this theoretical understanding.

The American public health physician, Avedis Donabedian, has worked for over 25 years on such a framework, which now forms the backbone of many quality initiatives in the USA and United Kingdom. He acknowledges the complexity of quality assessment, suggesting that only people who have 'not experienced the intricacies of clinical practice demand measures which are easy, precise and complete' (Donabedian 1988). However, he also suggests that attempts should be made to define and measure quality and that dividing it into three aspects, structure, process and outcome, can facilitate the process.

Structure. Structure relates to the setting in which care occurs. This includes consideration of facilities and amenities, equipment, money and human resources, such as the number and qualification of staff. It also relates to organisational issues such as management structures, methods of peer review and service levels. Thus, the structure or organisation of care determines some of its limits. Structures have fundamental effects on the care which can be offered to individual patients and the system in which care occurs determines to a large extent the processes available to health care staff.

Process. Process relates to the actual delivery of care and technical competence of the professional. The consumer's behaviour in seeking and complying with care is also included in this aspect. Donabedian clearly separates out two elements in the performance of practitioners, those of technical and interpersonal skill. The former relates to knowledge base and judgements used to decide on appropriate strategies of care, and skill in implementing these. He suggests that the quality of technical performance should be judged in comparison with the best in practice—that which is believed to produce the greatest improvement in health given current technology and knowledge. Williamson (1991) echoes this view, suggesting good professional performance occurs where practitioners are consistent in their treatment but seek to increase their knowledge of care options, and assess their advantages and cost effectiveness. Standards are set by the professionals them-selves as yardsticks against which to measure performance, and quality assurance programmes are designed to help them achieve the standards.

The interpersonal process is one by which technical care is implemented, and the success of the care depends upon it. The patient communicates the information needed for diagnosis, and the preferences necessary for selecting the most appropriate methods of care. The health professional in turn provides in-formation about the nature of the illness and its management and aims to motivate the patient to actively collaborate in care. The process is important since it must meet individual and social expectations and standards, such as privacy, confidentiality, in-formed choice, concern, empathy, honesty, tact and sensitivity. Donabedian suggests it is an aspect often ignored in quality assessment since it is not easy to measure or obtain information on. Yet interpersonal aspects of care are of considerable concern to patients, and processes of care may well affect outcome, as studies of the beneficial effects of placebos, for example, have shown. In addition, Smith & Cantley (1985) suggest that under-standing the process of care is very important if the objectives of various actors in the multidisciplinary setting are to be understood and the relationship between structures and outcomes explained.

Outcome. Outcome relates to the effectiveness of the service in terms of clinical results, patients' satisfaction with the care and its effect on health status, including improvements in patients' knowledge and changes in behaviour likely to bring about improved health. Of the three aspects, Donabedian sees outcomes as 'the ultimate validators of the effectiveness and quality of medical care' (Donabedian 1966, p. 169). He suggests that there is a scant understanding of the relationship between structural characteristics and processes of care but that the information which does exist indicates them to be weak and all that can accurately be said is whether conditions are conducive or unhelpful to good care.

Donabedian concludes that quality measurement is almost never carried out under the rigorous controls which scientific research requires and that most health-care evaluation relies on observational studies, where it is often impossible to directly attribute the observed outcomes to the process of care. Even with complex adjustments for case mix and other variables, the extent to which outcome is attributable to an antecedent process of care cannot be known for certain. He states:

'Quality assessment is neither clinical research nor technology assessment. It is primarily an administrative device used to monitor performance to determine whether it continues to remain within acceptable bounds.' (Donabedian 1988).

Williamson's (1991) comments on quality measurement suggest that structure is tangible and, so, can be assessed, and process can be determined to a large extent by protocol or practice guidelines. However, it is with outcome measures that problems occur since at present most are in their infancy or unable to be applied across the whole spectrum of care. Also, the degree to which a procedure is successful, not only in medical terms but also in its effect on the patients' well-being and their perceived health status, though important, is difficult to measure accurately with present techniques.

Returning to our original definition of a quality service:

one which meets consumer needs (or fulfils their expectation of it) as perceived by them and by the staff who work in the service

Donabedian acknowledges that patient satisfaction is a desired outcome of care, and that the subjective opinions of patients are valid and should be measured and the findings acted upon. Similarly, professional satisfaction should also be measured along with documentary evidence of service quality.

The audit of patient records checks that there has been access to and usage of resources and that key aspects of professional practice have been followed. Milne (1987) suggests that inadequate description of patient activity has been a notable problem in psychiatry. However, methods are now being developed to improve our understanding of the impact of certain programmes of care on patient or client functioning. As occupational therapists, if we hope our reports will be used by others in the multidisciplinary team to modify their method of providing care to ensure the client improves his task performance, then these reports must be of a sufficiently high standard to allow this to happen.

STANDARDS OF CARE

Preparing standards

The College of Occupational Therapists' (1989) definition of a standard is: 'an acceptable or approved example or statement of something against which measurement and/or judgement takes place; a level of quality relevant to the activity.'

Box 7.1 gives an example of such a standard.

Topic. The subject for a standard is usually prepared by identifying frequently occurring problems as stated by staff or patients, or concentrating on a particular area of operation such as admissions procedures or discharge arrangements. Standards are most often set by a group of staff working in the area under consideration, with or without managerial involvement. A system where standards are set and imposed 'from above' by those not in direct contact with the patients is not considered to be beneficial to involving all levels of staff in working towards the common goal of a high quality of care (Luthert & Robinson 1993).

Goal. A goal for the particular area must be set which is clear, specific and attainable, this may be set out as a sub-topic of the main standard.

Care group. A set of clients is then identified for whom the standard is to be written; this should be relevant to the whole group and to each member.

Standard statement. The standard statement is then prepared which is relevant to the topic, sub-topic and client group. It must be acceptable to all who will be using it and may require revisions before this is the case.

Criteria. The criteria specify the precise level of performance which has to be achieved in order to satisfy the standard. It is usually broken down into structure, process and outcome sub-criteria for further clarification.

Box 7.1   Example of a standard (adapted from Wright & Whittington 1992)

Topic: Patients on the Acute Admissions ward.
Sub-topic: Home assessment prior to discharge from the Acute Admissions ward.
Care group: All patients who are to be discharged into the community.
Standard statement: Each client will have a home assessment to prepare him or her for discharge and allow appropriate support services to be arranged if required.

Structure	Process	Outcome
Written departmental procedures on the protocol for home assessments	The OT identifies when a home visit is required within the treatment programme	The client has a comprehensive home assessment
A standardised home assessment form	The OT explains to the client and other relevant personnel the purpose of the home visit	The client is able to describe the care he requires on discharge
The necessary transport for a home visit available during working hours	The OT arranges the date and time of the home visit in consultation with the client, carers and other relevant personnel	On discharge, the client has a written copy of the agreed requirements arising from the home assessment
One qualified OT and one member of support staff available for each home assessment	The OT carries out a detailed daily living assessment with the client in the home environment	
	The OT identifies areas where intervention is required to allow maximum independence and safety on discharge	
	The OT discusses with the client, carers and support services methods of overcoming identified problem areas	
	The OT writes a full home assessment report detailing requirements prior to discharge	

Appraisal date: 9.11.93   Review date: 10.3.94   Authorised by: M Brown

- *Structural criteria* refer to the level of resource provision needed to achieve the standard.
- *Process criteria* specify the activities to be undertaken.
- *Outcome criteria* indicate the end results of care.

There are a large number of possible criteria and the standard setting group must choose those which are the best indicators and the easiest to use. Wright & Whittington (1992) suggest using the AMOUR principle to check the validity of each criterion—is it Achievable, Measurable, Observable, Understandable, and Reasonable?

Measuring standards

Once standards are set and agreed by all concerned with their measurement implications, techniques have to be selected which allow comparison between observed practice and the standard. The design of audit tools is an ongoing procedure and in the early stages of quality measurement it is useful to have a wide variety of measurement techniques in order to work out which are most sensitive and accurate for future use. Once the methods of appraisal are decided upon, a representative sample size is chosen which can be realistically handled.

Who carries out the appraisal?

The question of who appraises the standards is then raised—it may be the same group of people who have set them, on the grounds that they are most familiar with them, or it could be argued that this group should not do it since they are too close to the situation and may be biased towards a favourable outcome. Other possible appraisers are senior management, though professional staff may not welcome them in this role, so colleagues within a peer review group might be more acceptable as they have knowledge and expertise of the setting without being biased in favour of it, since it is not their own working area. Quality consultants from outside the NHS are sometimes used but they can be very expensive and may lack experience and understanding of the setting under consideration. Another group of appraisers could be members of a unit, district or trust audit committee. There might be members from the professional group, and clients or their representatives may be present as assessors.

In all these cases, a possible disadvantage is the feeling that any outside group cannot really understand what is occurring in a particular care setting.

Measurement techniques

Once these decisions have been made, measurement techniques may include the following, as appropriate to the standard being measured:

Simple observation. This is used for certain structural aspects; for example, are there the requisite number of fire hoses? Is there a chair for everyone waiting?

Direct observation. This is a useful method of concurrent appraisal of a standard where observers observe as it happens, but it is not without its difficulties in that those being observed may object and the observers must have sufficient experience to understand what is happening and make accurate observations.

Client notes or records audit. Here a group of staff randomly selects notes, examining what was done with the client and making suggestions for improvements. The audit team will be looking for such considerations as:

- Was the client correctly assessed according to his difficulty?
- Did the individual client plan address the issues identified?
- Was the client offered help to manage his own problems?
- Was the client provided with information about the ward/day hospital procedures and other relevant information?
- Were appropriate referrals made to other members of the multidisciplinary team?
- Was the client plan evaluated and changed as necessary?
- Was the presenting difficulty contained or resolved?

This method is only as good as the notes themselves and there may be a temptation to spend excessive time on notes to the detriment of patient care. An alternative method is to bring the case to a quality meeting which then suggests what could be done without knowing what was done in actuality. This may be a less threatening way to begin the process of quality audit in a department which has had little previous experience.

Satisfaction surveys. These are used with clients, relatives and staff, and come in numerous forms to suit the requirements of the standard, from large-scale questionnaires with computer analysed tick boxes to small-scale personal interviews.

Conferences and discussions. These occur with or without the patient/client and can yield useful information about all aspects of a standard area, rather than one small part. However, they are costly of the team's time, decisions may be difficult to pin down and bias may be introduced as a result of interpersonal relationships amongst the group or lack of objectivity about practice.

The auditing of a standard can be a lengthy and therefore costly procedure. A decision must be made, once the initial audit is complete, of how often the standard is to be reassessed. Yearly, or when a problem arises with some aspect of it, may be a realistic expectation.

Box 7.2 Calculating the observed compliance rate (adapted from Wright & Whittington 1992)

Topic: Patients on the Acute Admissions ward.
Sub-topic: Home assessment prior to discharge from the Acute Admissions ward.
Care group: All patients who are to be discharged into the community.
Standard statement: Each client will have a home assessment to prepare him or her for discharge and allow appropriate support services to be arranged if required.

Criteria	Measured by	Weighting	Yes	No
Has the client had a home visit?	Ask client Audit notes	50%	10	0
Is a detailed report available for distribution to other members of the team and support services?	Audit notes	20%	9	1
Can the client describe services required on discharge?	Client interview	20%	6	4
Does the client/carer have in writing the requirements identified by the home assessment?	Ask client/carer to show it	10%	9	1

Desired compliance rate = 95%

$$\text{Observed compliance rate} = \frac{(10 \times 50) + (9 \times 20) + (6 \times 20) + (9 \times 10)}{10}$$

$$= \frac{890}{10}$$

$$= 89\%$$

Comments: 10 patients appraised
1 Senior, 1 OT on sick leave

Assessor: J Green   Date: 9.11.93

Comparing appraisals

It is possible to arrive at a numerical indicator for how well or otherwise the standard has been met in order to compare it with future appraisals. Once the criteria have been set, as in Box 7.1, they can be worded in question form with the method of measurement identified (see Box 7.2). A weighting is given to each criterion indicating, in the opinion of the standard setters, its importance compared to the other criteria.

The number of patients who did or did not achieve the criteria is then set out in two columns of 'yes' or 'no'. The desired compliance rate will then be agreed as the acceptable percentage meeting the criteria for a high quality of service to be achieved.

The setting of this percentage is decided according to the type of standard. In the case of a fire procedure, for example, it would be desirous that all patients had the necessary knowledge, so a high quality of achievement of the standard would be 100%. However, other standards may be unlikely to reach that level and some other percentage, 85% for example, may be more realistic as an indicator of high quality.

The observed compliance rate is calculated at its simplest by:

$$\text{Observed compliance rate} = \frac{\text{Sum of (Weighting \% \times No. of 'yes')}}{\text{Sample size}}$$

Box 7.2 also illustrates a calculation of the applied compliance rate.

Once the information is collected, there must be a willingness on the part of all those involved to learn from any exposed shortcomings in the service. Well-set standards will throw up areas where practice is less than perfect, but standards which are set too low and expose nothing to work on towards improvement are a waste of time. Conversely, standards which are set impossibly high will lower morale and engender counterproductive feelings of hopelessness.

The concept of the improvement in quality as an ongoing process is apt, and quality efforts are often depicted as a wheel or spiral where standards are set, then appraised, planning followed by action results from the appraisal and so standards are reset in order to repeat the process (Fig. 7.1).

As already stated, quality monitoring can be expensive, but not as costly as failure to measure standards. This can lead to

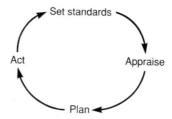

Figure 7.1 The quality wheel.

standards of care not being met, the client getting uncoordinated or duplicate services, less than efficient methods of treatment, unnecessary visits, tests or waiting times.

An obviously inefficient service can lower the morale and good-will among staff when practitioners are themselves disappointed in the service. Thus the cost of quality assurance initiatives should be outweighed by the savings of improved efficiency and effectiveness, along with client and staff satisfaction.

Towards good practice

Once we set out to define and measure the quality of care, there are implications for the managerial, educational and professional aspects of the service. Managers should be aware that there may be shown to be resource and budgetary implications in achieving high quality service. Whilst most health care settings are financially constrained, there must be sufficient flexibility to allocate or reallocate manpower, purchase some piece of equipment or send staff on an education programme.

Producing standards can act as an educational tool for new staff. Detailed standards are a guide to assessment, planning and implementing care, as well as its evaluation. They should also show to which members of the multidisciplinary team it is appropriate to refer clients. They can be used to define competency levels and ensure that the educational curricula of those in the service setting is appropriate to their need. Professionally, the standards define what each member of the team does in practice and can improve professional confidence and feelings of self-worth. They should ensure that there is no duplication of roles, which would not be cost effective, and that highly trained staff are not doing jobs for which they are overqualified. It is undoubtedly the case that multidisciplinary team work, in short-term psychiatric care, is greater than the sum of its parts and it is difficult to accurately attribute the efforts of an individual or professional group to the patients' care. It is important, however, as Wilson (1987) notes, for each member to define his or her own specialist input.

If quality assessment is to be a meaningful exercise, it must result in change for the better—for the patient, the staff who deliver care and the service as a whole. Quality of care research can inform our practice and save mistakes being made time and again. King et al (1971) found no direct link between staffing level and quality, although the allocation of more staff at peak activity periods, such as meal times and bed times is associated with more patient-centred care. Quality depends not on staff numbers but how they are organised and what they do. If staff are allocated to a small group of patients and remain with them through their day, then quality levels rise. If therapeutic interaction between staff and patients is important in treatment, then the percentage of time staff and patients interact together is important. Sanson-Fisher & Jenkins (1978) found staff interacting with patients for only 23% of their day and patients interacting only with other patients for 78% of theirs. Raynes et al (1979) looked at the size of an institution and the quality it offered and found that it is a high degree of autonomy within units, irrespective of institutional size, which contributes to a high quality of care. These examples serve to illustrate the importance of using the information brought to light by quality investigations to identify the reasons why there are differences between observed practice and the standards set.

The differences must be investigated and action plans to remedy them identified. Several options may be identified as possible solutions; it is up to the quality assurance group to select the best option, implement it and reappraise to check that it has brought about the improvement as hoped.

In cases where the observed practice has met or exceeds the standard, praise for the staff is important as a morale booster. However, where the observed practice is less good than the standard, the staff must be told specifically where shortfalls have occurred; this should be done in as positive and constructive way as possible. The feedback should be confidential.

Any action taken as a result of quality initiatives should be carefully thought through for all the possible solutions. These must be specific to the area of work or aspect of care which was identified and they must be realistic and acceptable to management and staff. Questions must be asked of all the alternative plans as to possible resource costs, time taken to achieve, effort required, implications for other parts of the system or unit.

Once an action plan is decided upon, it should be agreed by all involved with the project and specific guidelines drawn up to form a clear schedule of when each step should be carried out and the standard reappraised.

From time to time the standards group will review all the standards which have been set and operationalised. As time goes by, existing standards may be rewritten or new ones produced for new topics.

Maintaining quality is a continuing effort—conflict within the setting need not be bad if it is used positively to arrive at compromise solutions. Change requires time, effort and resources to support and sustain the process; it must be monitored and full explanations given to all involved. There needs to be an openness about quality improvement initiatives, so that the public, clients, relatives and interested others can see the efforts being made towards maximising the quality of patient or client care in the short-term psychiatric setting. No-one is suggesting that effecting change of this kind is easy, and psychiatric care has a difficult image to overcome at present as the large institutions close and some patients end up on the streets or in prison. If, as occupational therapists and members of the multidisciplinary team, we are to support the achievement of these high standards, then we shall have to work hard and be fully committed to them to achieve our aim.

As Ruskin said: 'Quality is never an accident; it is always the result of intelligent effort.'

REFERENCES

British Standards Institution 1987 BS5750 (ISO 9000 – 1987). British Standards Institution, Milton Keynes
College of Occupational Therapists 1989 Definitions relating to quality assurance. British Journal of Occupational Therapy 52(7): 270
Dean C et al 1993 Comparison of community based service with hospital based service for people with acute, severe psychiatric illness. British Medical Journal 307: 473–476
Department of Health 1962 The hospital plan for England and Wales. Cmnd 1604. HMSO, London
Department of Health 1989 Working for patients. Funding and contracts, working paper 2. HMSO, London

Department of Health 1990 Working for patients: operational principles. HMSO, London

Department of Health 1991 The Patients' Charter. HMSO, London

Department of Health and Social Security 1975 Better services for the mentally ill. Cmnd 6233. HMSO, London

Donabedian A 1966 Evaluating the quality of medical care. Millbank Memorial Fund Quarterly 44: 166–206

Donabedian A 1988 The quality of care—how can it be assessed? Journal of the American Medical Association 260(12): 1743–1748

Griffiths R 1983 NHS management inquiry report. DHSS, London

King R D et al 1971 Patterns of residential care. Routledge and Kegan Paul, London

Lavender A 1987 The measurement of the quality of care in psychiatric rehabilitation settings: development of the Model Standards Questionnaires. Behavioural Psychotherapy 15: 201–214

Luthert J, Robinson L (eds) 1993 The Royal Marsden Hospital manual of standards of care. Blackwell Scientific Publications, Oxford

Milne D 1987 Evaluating mental health practice. Croom Helm, Beckenham

Milne D, Learmonth M 1991 How to evaluate an occupational therapy service: a case study. British Journal of Occupational Therapy 54(2): 42–44

Moos R 1974 Evaluating treatment environments—a social ecological approach. Wiley, New York

National Health Service and Community Care Act 1990. HMSO, London

Ovretveit J 1990 What is quality in health services? Health Services Management (June): 132–133

Perkins R 1992 Do we measure up? The development of a multidisciplinary quality assurance and audit system in a psychiatric rehabilitation setting. Health Trends 24: 56–59

Pfeffer N 1992 Strings attached. Health Service Journal 2(April): 22–23

Raynes N V et al 1979 Organisational structure and the care of the mentally retarded. Croom Helm, London

Sanson-Fisher R, Jenkins H J 1978 Interaction patterns between in-mates and staff in a maximum security institution for delinquents. Behaviour Therapy 9: 703–716

Shepherd G 1984 Institutional care and rehabilitation. Longman, Harlow

Smith G, Cantley C 1985 Assessing health care. Open University Press, Milton Keynes

Social Services Committee 1988 The future of the NHS. 5th report. HMSO, London

Williamson J 1991 Providing quality care. Health Services Management (February): 18–23

Wilson C 1987 Hospital wide quality assurance: models for implementation and development. W B Saunders, Ontario

Wright C, Whittington D 1992 Quality assurance. An introduction for the health care professions. Churchill Livingstone, Edinburgh

PART 3

Intervention

8

Managing stress

Diana Keable

THE NATURE OF STRESS AND ANXIETY

Wherever occupational therapists offer their services, the demand for their skills in dealing with anxiety and stress-related problems is considerable. In acute mental health settings, this demand usually reaches its most urgent proportions. The effects and symptoms of anxiety and stress pervade the whole range of conditions encountered within the acute mental health field. Anxiety is a sprawling, insidious creature, and cannot be confined or contained within specific diagnostic categories. One of the reasons for this is that anxiety is a normal phenomenon; indeed it is essential to human survival and self-actualisation. It is only when an individual's anxiety rises beyond an adaptive level that it can be considered a clinical problem. The second reason is that we are all subject to external stresses over which we have a varying degree of control. Let us now differentiate between the terms 'stress' and 'anxiety'.

What is stress?

During the last two or three decades, it has become fashionable for the term 'stress' to be bandied about somewhat indiscriminately. Anxious individuals are frequently described as being in a 'state of stress', or even, more recently, 'stressed out'. In fact, stress, or

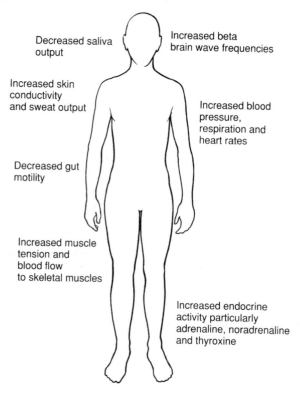

Decreased saliva output

Increased beta brain wave frequencies

Increased skin conductivity and sweat output

Increased blood pressure, respiration and heart rates

Decreased gut motility

Increased muscle tension and blood flow to skeletal muscles

Increased endocrine activity particularly adrenaline, noradrenaline and thyroxine

Figure 8.1 The fight/flight syndrome: activity in all major systems mobilised to cope with stress.

more properly, a stressor, is an external pressure which is brought to bear upon the individual (Selye 1976). That individual may, or may not, react to the stressor with an anxiety response. As we will see, each individual has a unique anxiety response pattern.

What is anxiety?

We have already said that anxiety is a normal human response to stress. Typically, it involves intense physiological arousal in order to prepare the individual for urgent physical and mental activity, i.e. the fight/flight syndrome. This manifests itself across several different systems simultaneously. Specifically, the brain, autonomic nervous system and endocrine system work together to produce this comprehensive response to stress (see Fig. 8.1).

While normal anxiety may serve to motivate individuals to improve their performance, neurotic anxiety generally has markedly negative effects. These include excessive physiological arousal, impaired cognitive performance and behavioural disruption. Sufferers of anxiety disorders may experience crippling levels of fear and emotional distress. The individual's self-esteem and confidence in his or her ability to cope with life's challenges is severely undermined (Keable 1989).

Anxiety disorders

Effects on health and function

- *Physiological*. Persistent physiological hyper-arousal, panic attacks, hyperventilation, psychosomatic conditions and pain.
- *Cognitive*. Impaired memory, concentration, task performance and decision-making skills, negative and irrational thinking, e.g. catastrophising, self-preoccupation.
- *Behavioural*. Avoidance of routine occupational tasks, e.g. shopping, travelling, going to work, as well as social and leisure activities. Illness behaviour, drug/alcohol abuse, marked dependence upon the support of others.
- *Emotional*. Fear, poor self-esteem, general emotional distress.

Fear response patterns

Sufferers of anxiety disorders invariably seek to reduce their fear and distress by avoiding the situations which intensify these feelings. A variety of reaction patterns may be adopted when an individual experiences an intense state of fear:

- fight/flight behaviour
- faint/freeze behaviour
- evasive/protective behaviour
- clinging behaviour/vocalisation of distress.

One or more of these behaviour patterns usually characterises the symptomatology in cases of neurotic anxiety.

State and trait anxiety

'State' anxiety may be described as a temporary condition involving subjective and physiological arousal. This is usually a relatively fleeting reaction to a stressful stimulus. 'Trait' anxiety, however, is a relatively enduring personality characteristic or tendency. People with strong trait anxiety tend to experience more frequent and intense anxiety states than the general population. They also tend to respond anxiously to a wider range of stimuli, which may include situations which are not generally considered particularly stressful, e.g. using public transport or shopping (Spielberger 1983).

Generalised and phobic anxiety

Anxiety may be a generalised or focused (phobic) condition. Generalised anxiety, sometimes called 'free-floating', involves a fairly persistent state of unease and tension. This may be punctuated by more marked episodes of state anxiety in response to stressful stimuli. Phobic anxiety is focused upon specific objects or situations which elicit the anxiety response, e.g. fear of spiders, lifts, open spaces. Very severe episodes of anxiety, i.e. panic attacks, are strongly associated with phobic anxiety. In practice, however, the distinction between generalised and phobic anxiety is seldom clear cut and clients frequently present with a rather muddy mixture of both.

Box 8.1 Predisposing and current factors in the aetiology of anxiety disorders

Predisposing factors
- Temperament: inherited traits
- Early psychological trauma, particularly disrupted mother–child relationship
- Stressful life events during maturation, particularly separation
- Exposure to unfavourable environment during maturation, e.g. poor housing, lack/surfeit of stimulation, growing up in a deprived institutional environment or a war zone
- Basic physical needs unmet: hunger/cold
- Faulty learning of maladaptive coping styles

Current factors
- Stressful life events, e.g. bereavement, giving birth, relocation, unemployment, legal/criminal activity
- Stressful lifestyles: conflictual roles, e.g. 'working mother', financial problems, study/work-related pressure
- Social stress: role dissatisfaction/ambiguity, poor social status, poverty, poor accommodation
- Relationship/family problems, e.g. divorce, caring for sick relatives or children
- Actual/potential physical ill health, especially terminal/progressive illness of self/significant other

Aetiological factors in anxiety disorders

The aetiology of anxiety disorders is a wide-ranging and complex subject area. The effects of a variety of predisposing factors interact with current influences (Box 8.1) to bring about a unique clinical picture in each sufferer.

Thus, the aetiology of anxiety may be approached from various different schools of thought:

- Physiological
- Cognitive–behavioural
- Psycho-dynamic
- Sociological.

The basic tenets relating to anxiety from these different theoretical perspectives have been described in more depth elsewhere (Beck & Emery 1985, Keable 1989, Levitt 1980, Sims & Snaith 1988).

THE MANAGEMENT OF ANXIETY

The following list gives examples from the vast array of approaches that may be offered as legitimate interventions in the treatment of anxiety:

- alternative medicine, including aromatherapy, acupuncture, homeopathy, massage, herbal medicine and various dietary regimes
- chemotherapy
- cognitive therapy
- counselling/psychotherapy
- exercise therapy
- life skills techniques, e.g. assertiveness training, goal-setting and problem-solving techniques
- relaxation training
- yoga.

The treatment of choice selected here is 'anxiety management training'. This is a comprehensive approach which contains many elements from the above list. It was developed in accordance with the cognitive–behaviour modification model (Meichenbaum 1977, Suinn & Richardson 1971). Anxiety management programmes may be adapted to meet widely diverging needs. For example, graded, practical programmes may be developed for those with learning/memory disabilities. Alternatively, stress management programmes for business executives are increasingly popular, focusing on occupational stress, time management and problem-solving skills. The programme outlined here is more suitable for clients with a clinical anxiety disorder, who might be expected to require treatment in an acute mental health setting.

Rationale

Anxiety management training emphasises the need to develop self-control skills in order to cope effectively with both cognitive and physiological arousal. The learning of effective coping skills is held to extinguish the need to respond maladaptively to stressful situations. The cognitive–behavioural modification model describes anxiety as a multidimensional problem and attempts to deal with symptoms on several levels simultaneously. Thus, anxiety management programmes are aimed at the replacement of ineffective coping responses with an array of positive strategies or coping skills. Clients are encouraged to achieve personal control or self-mastery over their own symptoms.

Training regimes involve three basic components: education, skills acquisition and skills application.

Education. This aspect involves teaching clients accurate facts about stress, and their physical and mental responses to it. The emphasis is upon dispelling inaccurate, often alarming, notions about the meaning of anxiety symptoms. Clients frequently mis-label signs of anxiety such as hyperventilation, believing that such symptoms indicate serious physical illness or impending death.

Skills acquisition. A variety of physical and mental coping skills including relaxation techniques and positive, rational thinking strategies may be taught. This ensures that clients are armed with a range of techniques to choose from to assist them in coping with different situations. Thus, individual variations in need, ability and preference among different clients are allowed for.

Skills application. Throughout training, the client is expected to take responsibility for practising the techniques and applying them to cope with problems outside the session. This may include the use of homework assignments, stress diaries and self-rating scales. Goal-setting and problem-solving techniques may be used to assist the clients in achieving their personal objectives.

Box 8.2 provides a suggested format for an eight-module anxiety management course.

Box 8.2   An eight-module anxiety management course

Module 1
- Introduce general concepts relating to anxiety and stress, e.g. fight/flight syndrome, effects of avoidance.
- Demonstrate 'contrast relaxation' to facilitate muscle tension awareness (see 'Techniques').

Module 2
- Focus on biological concepts relating to physical signs and symptoms of anxiety, including hyperventilation.
- Describe characteristic stress postures, rationale of muscle relaxation techniques and how exercise fits in.
- Group exercise to test for muscle tension in pairs (Marquis et al 1980).
- Group exercise: demonstrate 'loosening up' exercises to disperse muscle tension and restlessness before relaxation.
- Teach 'simple relaxation' (Mitchell 1977).

Module 3
- Discuss differential/applied relaxation and advise on how to use relaxation skills in everyday activities (Mitchell 1977). Emphasise need to recognise early warning signs of escalating anxiety.
- Group exercise: brainstorm different stressful situations and ways of coping.
- Demonstrate differential techniques, i.e. methods of standing, walking, sitting and doing a simple task in a relaxed manner, using only essential levels of muscle tension (Keable 1989).
- Teach 'emergency' relaxation techniques, emphasising breathing management.

Module 4
- Give short, irrational beliefs test, e.g. Ellis (Ellis & Harper 1972). Score and discuss.
- Describe concepts and types of faulty (irrational) thinking, e.g. catastrophising, global thinking, unreasonable assumptions/expectations of self/others (Ellis & Harper 1972, Beck et al 1974).
- Using examples from client group, examine causes and effects of negative thinking styles, e.g. 'I can't cope'.
- Teach use of positive thinking and methods of challenging irrational beliefs.
- Teach mental relaxation techniques, e.g. Benson's 'relaxation response' and visualisation (Benson 1976).

Module 5
- Reinforce recognition of, and ability to challenge, faulty thinking in stressful situations.
- Group exercise: discuss and challenge individual examples of faulty thinking.
- Discuss stressful life events and difficulties associated with change.
- Discuss the mechanisms of avoidance behaviour in reinforcing anxiety.
- Visualisation: imaginal rehearsal of three stressful situations within session (see 'Techniques').

Module 6
- Teach goal-setting methods; assist clients to set realistic personal goals and break them down into specific, realistic behavioural targets.
- Teach problem-solving technique.

- Group exercise: select one client example and work through problem-solving process within the session (Keable 1989).

Module 7
- Discuss social needs and difficulties, e.g. leisure outlets, work roles, relationships.
- Teach basic principles of social skills, including nonverbal and verbal behaviour (Hewitt 1988).
- Managing your anxiety while using assertiveness techniques.
- Role play client examples of problematic social situations.

Module 8
- Group exercise: give revision test, score, and discuss results.
- Revise and reinforce main points covered throughout course.
- Continue and complete individual role play examples.
- Discuss how to consolidate achievements post-course and explain follow-up arrangements.

Techniques

A brief overview of the anxiety-reduction techniques that are used as part of the anxiety management course is given here.

Contrast relaxation

Commonly mislabelled 'progressive' relaxation, this technique is probably the most widely used of all relaxation methods. The technique is characterised by its use of deliberate and exaggerated tensing or clenching of muscles, followed by releasing or 'letting go'. This mostly involves the flexor or antagonist groups of muscles. True 'progressive' relaxation, as described by Jacobsen (1938), is a much more thorough and complex procedure, which may take months to learn. The main advantage of contrast relaxation is that it facilitates recognition of the difference between tension and relaxation. Its main drawback is that clients are frequently unable to let go of the tension created, thus compounding the state of tension (Keable 1989).

Simple relaxation

Designed by Mitchell (1977), a physiotherapist, this technique is to be highly recommended for basic physiological relaxation. It is simple to learn and teach and can be adapted for use in most clinical settings. Commands are given for movements of the agonist muscle groups only, so that the body is moved out of stereo-typical stressed postures, and into relaxed ones. For example, 'pull your shoulders down'. The technique is based on sound physiological principles, i.e. reciprocal inhibition, although few published outcome studies of its use in this clinical setting exist.

Differential/applied relaxation

This group of techniques refer to 'relaxation in action'. It is essential that relaxation training is not presented merely as a passive process. Once the basic methods of muscle relaxation have been taught, clients should progress to using them actively, and in different situations, i.e. sitting, standing, walking and carrying out tasks (Keable 1989). Key positions should be developed which are used to prompt generalised relaxation during activity (Mitchell 1977). These may be linked to emergency relaxation and breathing control techniques for use in panic management.

The relaxation response

Essentially, this technique is based on the practice of meditation. However, it is a clinically standardised form of meditation and contains no religious or mystical element (Benson 1976). It includes the use of a neutral focal device—usually the silent repetition of a word of the client's choosing. This technique has great potential in helping clients to gain control over anxious thinking patterns. However, in the initial stages of training, many clients find considerable difficulty in concentrating for long enough to derive much benefit from this technique.

Visualisation

The use of visualisation is becoming increasingly widespread in psychological and general medicine, orthodox and otherwise, e.g. holistic cancer regimes, pain management. It is, of course, an infinitely flexible and powerful technique which can be applied creatively to meet the needs of a particular individual or group. For those suffering from psychotic conditions, its use is contra-indicated. This is because visualisation involves elements of suggestion and fantasy which may compound psychotic symptoms. Care should also be taken not to encourage dependence on the therapist by too much emphasis on therapist-led visualisation, as in guided fantasy journeys.

In the context of anxiety management, clients can be taught to use visualisation to gain independent control over their symptoms. For example, visualisation can be used to rehearse feared situations imaginally, thus bringing about a degree of desensitisation prior to exposure. It may also be used to assist in deepening relaxation in a variety of ways, e.g. imagine the muscles softening and lengthening as they relax.

Notes on presentation

Setting

The training environment should be comfortably warm, well ventilated and with sufficient floor space to allow the use of relaxation mats. The room should afford some privacy but need not be darkened or kept absolutely free from extraneous noise. A realistic environment helps clients to learn to relax in less than ideal conditions. The availability of supportive chairs, pillows and mats is more important.

Session length and frequency

As a general guide, at least an hour and a half is usually required to allow adequate time to cover the material for each of the suggested modules. Alternatively, the material may be covered over two or more briefer sessions. This format is more suitable for clients with shorter concentration spans.

It is generally convenient to hold sessions once weekly, and this allows time for practice and consolidation of skills between sessions. Where a shorter, more intensive course structure is required, sessions could be held twice weekly. A more relaxed pace could be offered by covering the same material over a longer period of time.

As the above demonstrates, the length and frequency of sessions are infinitely adaptable according to the learning needs of the client group being treated.

Group training formats

Anxiety management is generally presented in a course format, i.e. over a certain number of weeks, within the context of a closed group. This format is probably the ideal method but is often beset by a number of practical problems. Firstly, sufficient numbers of suitable clients have to be gathered and interviewed well in advance. A waiting list has to be set up and the course advertised to referring agencies. For staff involved, a considerable amount of planning and administration is therefore required. For clients in urgent need of this kind of help, a lengthy wait for the course to start may be unacceptable.

A possible alternative is to set up a rolling programme on an open group basis, so that clients may enter the course as soon as they are referred. This may mean starting at week four or seven, for example, and continuing until all the sessions have been covered. This format also allows clients to repeat sessions if necessary. However, greater flexibility may be gained at the cost of group cohesiveness. Cohesiveness, along with attendant motivational benefits, is likely to be greater for the closed group format.

Individual clients

Clients may be treated very successfully on an individual basis where circumstances dictate, for example in the client's own home. However, the effectiveness of anxiety management training is generally enhanced by being applied within a group context. This is because clients learn a great deal from each other's experiences, not least the realisation that 'they are not alone'. In a cohesive group, clients support and encourage each other to achieve their goals, as well as bringing peer pressure to bear when required.

Session structure

Sessions may be divided into the following sections:

1. Feedback from client's homework practice
2. Educational topics, e.g. 'fight/flight syndrome', irrational thinking, principles of goal-setting/problem-solving
3. Skill learning, e.g. various relaxation techniques
4 Short concluding feedback, clarifying homework required for next session.

Over-long periods devoted solely to relaxation are generally unrealistic and unhelpful as they engender dependence on the therapist.

Teaching accessories

Various tools exist which the therapist may use to illuminate the message and enhance the client's retention and understanding:

- books and handouts
- visual aids
- tapes.

The provision of reading material, such as handouts, is an invaluable way of reinforcing the material covered within sessions. This allows clients to consolidate and expand their knowledge of the topic as well as catch up on any sessions missed. The use of visual aids serves to clarify concepts covered during the sessions, particularly when unfamiliar or complex ideas are being discussed, such as the mechanics of hyperventilation, or problem-solving strategies. Many therapists will already be familiar with the use of overhead projectors and flip charts. The writer also finds the humble blackboard and chalks indispensable, particularly for brainstorming sessions.

However, there are inherent pitfalls associated with the use of audio-taped relaxation instructions. The first, and most serious, of these is the danger of creating dependence. It is crucial that clients learn to relax in response to their own internally generated cues. Tapes can interfere with this process, and may also serve to limit generalisation of skills. Secondly, it has been known for some time that 'live' relaxation training is superior to taped instruction (Paul & Trimble 1970, Lehrer & Woolfolk 1993). As a general rule, it is probably wisest to avoid using tapes altogether. However, those with exceptional difficulties in memorising the instructions may be helped to overcome this with relaxation tapes. It is suggested that they are only used in the initial learning phase and withdrawn as swiftly as possible. Rather than recording her own voice, the therapist could suggest that clients make their own relaxation tapes.

Homework

It should be emphasised in the strongest possible terms that independent practice of coping skills is crucial. Quite simply, if the clients fail to practice the techniques, then they must expect meagre benefits. Engaging the clients' commitment to this is the therapist's most important task in anxient management. All too frequently, it will also be the therapist's most difficult task! Before moving on to suggest some helpful strategies for achieving this end, it is necessary to look at what kind of homework to set.

Relaxation techniques. Practice of a simple and effective muscle relaxation technique such as the Mitchell method (1977) should be advised on a daily basis for 10- to 20-minute periods. These can be adjusted to fit in with the client's individual lifestyle.

Written homework. This is given in order to consolidate the material covered in the preceding session, or to prepare for topics to be covered in the next session. Examples may include lists of personal 'early warning signs' of mounting tension, negative self-statements/stress triggers, personal goals and problems, relevant questionnaires.

Action-based assignments. These should be related to each client's personal goals and will often involve carrying out dreaded, and previously avoided, activities such as shopping expeditions, telephone calls, returning to work, interviews or social events.

Suggested strategies for ensuring that client homework is done

- Create an expectation that homework is an essential requirement and explain why.
- Agree individual/group-based contracts about non-completion of homework.
- Start each session with feedback from clients' homework.
- Use self-rating scales and individual graphs/charts to monitor and reinforce progress.
- Provide flexible and realistic advice for clients who encounter difficulties in independent practice.
- Set homework tasks that are appropriate in nature and pace for the client/group being treated.
- Always be assiduous in following up any default on homework.

It is vital to establish and reinforce the expectation that clients should do homework as part of the course. The need for the client to take responsibility for the outcome of treatment must be emphasised at all times. Ideally, the client's agreement to this should be obtained prior to commencement. This may be done in the form of an individual or group contract, agreed mutually between the therapist and the client/s. For example, such a contract might state that treatment will be terminated and reviewed if the client defaults on three consecutive homework assignments. It should be pointed out that anxiety management is a teaching technique and that once the skills have been taught it is up to the client to put them into practice.

Naturally, the therapist expects to encounter motivational deficits. It is usually best to acknowledge that many clients will not find independent practice easy, especially at first, but that the ultimate benefits are great. The therapist's approach must, of course, be sensitive, but firm. Clients frequently experience particular difficulties in using relaxation techniques. They may complain of being distracted by worrying thoughts, or difficulty in finding time to practice or in overcoming incorrect breathing habits. The therapist must try to help clients to find realistic and creative solutions to these problems. This process is facilitated by inviting other group members to share their experiences and make suggestions.

It is essential to start each session with feedback from homework. Homework sheets which incorporate 'before and after' self-rating scales should be used as the basis for this. These have the dual advantage of measuring progress as well as providing a motivating factor. Data from daily self-rating scales may also be collated over a period of weeks and transferred to a personal progress graph/chart. In this way, clients are able to see the gradual improvements they have made over time.

In group sessions, peer pressure can be exploited to good advantage. Excuses such as 'I didn't have time' or 'I was too stressed/too little stressed' can be respectfully but firmly dealt with as teaching points. Examples of good progress gained as a result of assiduous practice can also be highlighted.

Action-based assignments will usually be tackled towards the end of the course when the client has acquired some proficiency in using the relevant coping skills. Care should be exercised in the timing and pacing of these assignments in order to avoid loss of confidence, especially where exposure to a feared situation is involved. Goal-setting methods should be used in order to break down the assignment into graded, manageable targets, thus facilitating increasing self-mastery.

Selection criteria

As we have already highlighted, the selection criteria for anxiety management training may be fairly broad because the technique can be adapted to suit the client/client group. It should be acknowledged that most psychiatric conditions, and indeed many physical ones, are complicated by a significant element of anxiety. Frequently, however, anxiety is the most distressing factor for clients presenting with depressive illness, adjustment crises and even some psychotic disorders.

However, certain contraindications apply. Relaxation training and related techniques should not be used with those suffering from florid psychosis or acute mania. In the case of psychosis, the ability to discriminate fantasy from reality may be impaired. Techniques using visualisation or guided fantasy, in particular, are likely to exacerbate symptoms. In the case of acute mania, disinhibited behaviour is likely to disrupt the client's ability to engage with the technique, especially in a group situation. The following groups also present temporary or permanent difficulties which may preclude or limit potential to benefit from this technique:

- disruptive/disturbed behaviour
- substantial cognitive skills deficits, e.g. advanced dementia, severe brain injuries
- substantial verbal skills deficits
- excessive state anxiety.

It is recommended that screening guidelines be issued to referring agencies in order to eliminate inappropriate referrals.

Assessment

This is as vital a part of anxiety management training, as it is in every other clinical intervention used by occupational therapists (Finlay 1988, Creek 1990). Some of the aims relevant here are:

- to provide accurate and comprehensive information about the problems and needs presented
- to assist both client and therapist in setting up realistic goals of treatment
- to guide the selection of appropriate treatment techniques
- to measure the extent of the problem before, during and after treatment so that change can be identified
- to provide data for treatment outcome evaluation and research.

Anxiety is a multifactorial phenomenon. Therefore a single-pronged approach may not be sufficient to ensure comprehensive assessment. Instead, it may be useful to consider anxiety in terms of five interacting elements, i.e. physiological, cognitive, social, behavioural and subjective/emotional. Some of these elements may be measured in a reasonably straightforward manner, others are very difficult to assess objectively. The decision about which data-gathering tools/procedures to use may be guided by the following considerations:

- the needs and abilities of the client group, e.g. verbal skills, clients' goals
- the envisaged nature and extent of the problem/s
- the constraints of the clinical setting, e.g. time available, staff training required
- the ultimate purpose of the assessment, whether routine clinical or research related.

Some brief notes on the types of assessments that may be used in anxiety management training

1. Interview procedures using internally devised, structured schedules/questionnaires.
2. Structured observation methods, e.g. behavioural observation, role play trials.
3. Physical examinations, e.g. skin temperature, pulse and respiration rates.
4. Standardised assessment tools/psychometric tests, e.g. the State–Trait Anxiety Inventory (Spielberger 1983).

The first two assessment methods are primarily designed to collect *qualitative* information. These methods are fairly flexible but can be tailored to meet specific information collection requirements. Of all the assessment methods, questionnaires and interview schedules are probably the most common and easiest to use. However, these approaches frequently suffer from design inadequacies which may distort the quality of information collected. Structured observations require some careful thought at the planning and setting-up stage. Various forms of technology may be employed to assist in the process. The two main advantages of this approach are first that the client is involved actively, and secondly that treatment events are recorded in a precise manner.

The latter two groups listed are primarily designed to collect *quantitative* information. Their main advantage is that they are much more objective and demonstrably accurate than qualitative approaches. Great caution must be exercised, however, when physical examinations are used, to select reliable and appropriate techniques of measurement. Many extraneous factors can affect the reliability of the data, e.g. heart/respiration rates affected by time of day/last meal and who/what is carrying out the measurement.

Standardised tests depending on the use of interval data (i.e. data which follow the normal frequency distribution curve) which have been properly validated are underused in the clinical situation. They are essential for clinical research so that outcomes can be compared with those of similar studies. Their ease of use varies widely according to the test selected. Standardised tests often suffer from rigidity in their application, and many require specific training to administer. All the methods of assessment noted here have already been described in greater detail elsewhere (Keable 1989).

Evaluation

The quality of treatment evaluation depends on the accuracy and thoroughness of the assessment method employed. However, overburdened therapists often find it difficult to put time aside to develop improved assessment and evaluation procedures. Despite this very real problem, attention paid to these issues can result in both improved treatment quality for the client; and hard data to support arguments to protect/increase resources.

With this in mind, therapists should strive to regularly and systematically collect data about treatment outcomes. Appropriately designed clinical audit procedures may assist in emphasising qualitative aspects of outcome rather than mere volume of clients treated. In the case of anxiety management training, data should be collected before and after treatment and again at the follow-up stage to record change over a longer period.

Discontinuing treatment

For those on training courses of a predetermined length, the question of when to stop treatment is answered clearly from the start. For those on a rolling programme, especially where there has been a disappointing response to training, the answer may not be so easy. Part of the answer lies in ensuring that clear, realistic goals of treatment are set up before commencement, and agreed with the client. This is especially crucial for more flexible, individualised treatment delivery formats. Progress should then be monitored throughout treatment and its ultimate outcome measured objectively (see 'Assessment'). The therapist and client will then have collected sufficient evidence to decide which of the following apply:

- The client has achieved none or unacceptably few of her goals.
- The client has achieved all or most of her goals.
- The client has consistently failed to attend treatment sessions or complete homework assignments.

In any of the above scenarios, it is counterproductive for the client to continue endlessly in training. Instead, other options which may better suit the client's needs should be explored. Obviously, some clients are genuinely working at their problems but need longer to reach their goals.

Follow-up

Having access to follow-up greatly assists the client in taking steps towards true independence in anxiety management. Many clients view their discharge with far less trepidation, in the knowledge that they have a follow-up appointment. Short-term follow-up appointments are often set at 4–6 weeks post-course, and long-term follow-up may take place from 4–12 months post-course. Assessment procedures can be repeated at each follow-up appointment in order to evaluate progress and the maintenance of skills.

PROBLEMS, PITFALLS, AND SOME USEFUL STRATEGIES

Prevention is better than cure

At the outset, the therapist should ensure that:

- the approach used is suited to the needs and abilities of the client/client group in question
- the presentation and training content is of a high standard
- the approach used does not actively foster client dependence on the therapist
- the primary aim is to facilitate application of the skills to a client's individual problems and lifestyle *outside* the clinical situation.

Why isn't the treatment working?

When problems do occur it is important to identify, as accurately as possible, what the likely causes are. Some of the most frequent reasons for lack of success in learning/using self-help anxiety reduction methods include:

- poor motivation
- external 'locus of control' (Sandler & Lakey 1982, Seligman 1975)
- client dependence on therapist
- cognitive problems, e.g. poor concentration
- lack of application outside clinical setting
- poor independent practice rates
- excessive acute/state anxiety
- florid psychotic symptoms/acute behavioural disturbance
- side effects of medication, e.g. muscle rigidity/motor restlessness/drowsiness
- negative feelings/attitudes towards the therapist, e.g. hostility, scepticism
- external agents such as drug treatments which the client deems more credible than self-help methods
- use of muscle tension as a psychological defence mechanism resulting in a fear of relaxation
- need to maintain symptoms for various psycho-dynamic reasons, e.g. to meet dependency needs
- staff-related problems, e.g. lack of continuity/expertise.

The therapist will need to use his or her skills in assessment and evaluation in order to identify the problems hindering the individual client's progress. Once this stage has been reached, the therapist should then be in a better position from which to recommend an appropriate action plan. Broadly, this may involve one of the following options:

- Discontinue/delay treatment: this may involve discharging the client, and/or referring to an alternative agency/treatment approach.
- Adapt treatment to meet the client's needs more effectively and enable the client to overcome obstacles.

In nearly every case, the therapist should avoid allowing the client to continue aimlessly in on-going treatment. The problem-solving process must be applied in each individual case. Failure to act positively will result in the demoralisation of both client and therapist.

Preventive strategies

Develop an adequate screening procedure to avoid inappropriate referrals. Clients should not be accepted for treatment if they are unlikely to benefit, or do not see it as relevant to their problems.

Clarify what the client may expect from treatment, before it commences. The more accurate the clients' expectation of treatment, the more likely they are to be satisfied with it, and motivated to participate. It is vital to explain the self-help emphasis of the techniques, and also to enumerate the benefits that may be gained, e.g. the ability to control distressing anxiety symptoms independently, increased confidence and self-esteem.

Clarify your expectations of the client before treatment. Gain the client's agreement, if necessary, by establishing a treatment contract. The therapist should aim to negotiate terms that the clients themselves consider fair. For example, it is sometimes appropriate to inform clients that they will be suspended from treatment, pending review, if they repeatedly default on attendance or fail to complete a sufficient number of homework assignments. The nature of the strategies employed will, of course, depend on the needs of the client/client group in question. It is crucial that treatment expectations of clients are realistic in the first place so as not to set the client up for failure, and further demotivation.

Present high-quality training sessions. Sessions should be well prepared, interesting and relevant to clients' needs. The course should aim to provide an empowering experience which fully involves the clients whom it is attempting to reach. Therapists should acknowledge the value of the clients' contribution to the therapeutic process.

Make clients' homework assignments the most important part of the training process. Use every appropriate tool to achieve this, e.g. regular homework feedback sessions, daily practice self-rating scales, personal progress log books, intermittent graphs of personal progress, peer pressure, treatment contracts, positive reinforcement from therapist (see 'Homework').

Phase out therapist's leadership role as rapidly as possible. The techniques, e.g. relaxation, usually need to be demonstrated once or twice only. The emphasis should then be placed on client-centred feedback about practice of skills and progress outside the clinical setting.

Present relaxation techniques in a manner that does not reinforce dependence on the therapist. Some common pitfalls of this kind are:

- Speaking in soft, soothing tones when teaching relaxation. Clients often enjoy this so much that they never learn to relax without the therapist's gentle voice to lead them!
- Insisting that relaxation shoud be carried out in dimly lit, absolutely silent environments. This is not realistic—clients must eventually learn to relax in highly stressful situations.
- Failing to encourage clients to vary the postures/situations in which they practice, i.e. relaxation may be carried out when sitting, lying, standing and walking.
- Teaching only one, or a limited range, of relaxation techniques. Anxious clients need an armoury of strategies for use in a variety of situations.
- Failing to encourage clients to move on and advance their skill levels. Training should be organised progressively.

Enable clients to set specific, realistic goals related to the problems they are experiencing. Encourage clients to apply the skills that they have learned to tackle real problems and improve their lifestyle outside the clinical setting. They should set concrete, achievable targets so that improvements can be readily identified.

Discharge clients at an appropriate stage in their treatment. It is better to discharge clients rather than create the additional problem of dependence. Clients with residual problems can be offered a course of follow-up sessions, aimed at empowering them to deal with remaining problems independently (see 'Discontinuing treatment').

REFERENCES

Beck A T, Emery G 1985 Anxiety disorders and phobias. Basic Books, New York
Beck A T, Laude R, Bohnert M 1974 Ideational components of anxiety neurosis. Archives of General Psychiatry 31: 319–325
Benson H 1976 The relaxation response. Collins, London
Creek J 1990 Occupational therapy and mental health: principles, skills and practice. Churchill Livingstone, Edinburgh

Ellis A, Harper R A (eds) 1972 A guide to rational living. Wilshire, North Hollywood

Finlay L 1988 Occupational therapy practice in psychiatry. Chapman & Hall, London

Hewitt C 1988 Training in social skills. In Willson M (ed) Occupational therapy in short-term psychiatry, 2nd edn. Churchill Livingstone, Edinburgh

Jacobsen E 1938 Progressive relaxation, 2nd edn. University Press, Chicago

Keable D 1989 The management of anxiety—a manual for therapists. Churchill Livingstone, Edinburgh

Lehrer P M, Woolfolk R L 1993 Principles and practice of stress management, 2nd edn. Guilford Press, New York

Levitt E E 1980 The psychology of anxiety, 2nd edn. Lawrence Erlbaum, Hillside, NJ

Marquis J N, Ferguson J M, Barr Taylor C 1980 Generalization of relaxation skills. Journal of Behaviour Therapy and Experimental Psychiatry 11: 95–99

Meichenbaum D 1977 Cognitive behaviour modification. Plenum Press, New York

Mitchell L 1977 Simple relaxation. John Murray, London

Paul G L, Trimble R W 1970 Recorded vs 'live' relaxation training and hypnotic suggestion. Comparative effectiveness for reducing physiological arousal and inhibiting stress responses. Behaviour Therapy 1: 285–302

Sandler I N, Lakey B 1982 Locus of control as a stress moderator: the role of control perceptions and social support. American Journal of Community Psychology 102: 187–193

Seligman M E P 1975 Helplessness. Freeman, San Francisco

Selye H 1976 Stress in health and disease. Butterworth, Massachusetts

Sims A, Snaith P 1988 Anxiety in clinical practice. John Wiley, Chichester

Spielberger C D 1983 Manual for the state–trait anxiety inventory (Form Y). Consulting Psychologists Press, California

Suinn R M, Richardson F 1971 Anxiety management training: a non-specific behaviour therapy program for anxiety control. Behaviour Therapy 2: 498–510

FURTHER READING

Beck A T, Emery G 1985 Anxiety disorders and phobias. Basic Books, New York

Beech H R, Burns L E, Sheffield B F 1982 A behavioural approach to the management of stress: a practical guide to techniques. John Wiley, Chichester

Benson H 1976 The relaxation response. Collins, London

Cullen B 1988 The management of anxiety. In: Willson M (ed) Occupational therapy in short-term psychiatry, 2nd edn. Churchill Livingstone, Edinburgh

Grings W W, Dawson M E 1978. Emotions and bodily responses: a psycho-physiological approach. Academic Press, Chicago

Keable D 1989. The management of anxiety—a manual for therapists. Churchill Livingstone, Edinburgh

Kennerley H 1989 Managing anxiety: a training manual. Oxford University Press, Oxford

Lehrer P M, Woolfolk R L 1993 Principles and practice of stress management, 2nd edn. Guilford Press, New York

Levitt E E 1980 The psychology of anxiety, 2nd edn. Lawrence Erlbaum, Hillside, NJ

Meichenbaum D 1985 Stress inoculation training. Allyn, USA

Miller R J, Cullen B, O'Brien R 1981 Are you sitting comfortable? Psychological approaches to the management of stress and anxiety. Occupational Therapy 44(1): 5–9

Mitchell L 1977 Simple relaxation. John Murray, London

Richards S C 1978 When self-control fails: a case study of the maintenance problem in self-control treatment programs. Cognitive Therapy and Research 2(4): 397–401

Sims A, Snaith P 1988 Anxiety in clinical practice. John Wiley, New York

9

Creative therapies

Barbara Steward

INTRODUCTION

There is no intention in this chapter to replicate guidelines and exercise manuals which are comprehensively available elsewhere. The aim here is to review and reflect on the use of creative therapies and the controversies which surround what should be done, to whom, by which therapists, to what end, now and in the future.

Although creative therapies are a relatively recent addition to the repertoire of the occupational therapist, the notion that artistic expression has curative and palliative effects on the mentally ill is far from new. Initially, the main therapeutic emphasis was on the soothing and civilising effect of art itself. Then, as psychiatry moved from custodial to curative care, and the work of psycho-analysts and humanists became increasingly influential, the creativity assumed a more central position in the treatment of the mentally ill (Busuttil 1990).

The use of specific creative therapies increased in response to a number of forces.

• The dramatic evolution in chemotherapy enabled psychiatric staff to move away from behavioural control to facilitating behavioural change.
• Employment of patients in hospital agriculture and industries was no longer considered appropriate, so activities geared to the maintenance of the institution were replaced by rehabilitation.

- Medication controlled acute symptoms so that patients could participate in action and talking therapies.
- The influence of analytic and humanist models of psychiatry in the UK, rather than the predominant behaviourist approach of the USA, established an environment where creative therapies could flourish.
- The 1960s and 1970s witnessed the development of therapeutic communities and therapeutic milieux where group therapy and creative self-expression became the predominant treatment approaches.
- Changes in public attitudes to psychiatric illness, and greater understanding of causes and treatments, increased the acceptance of dynamic, group psychotherapies.

There has always been disagreement about the origins of creative therapies. Some therapists identify their roots in the arts, others in psychiatry and others in rehabilitation. Ownership and rights to practice often lie at the roots of this debate.

There were parallel evolutions to creative therapy, with art and drama specialists adapting and developing techniques for use in health care, while creative group work was added to occupational therapy courses.

WHAT ARE CREATIVE THERAPIES?

There are considerable problems in clumping together all the creative therapies and discussing them as a single entity and doing so will inevitably create some unacceptable generalisations. However, these techniques do share some of the following common goals, approaches and philosophies:

- The participants need no specific artistic skill.
- The process of creating is more important than the creative product.
- The activities are generally cooperative not competitive.
- Through the process of being creative, the participants experience emotions and new understandings about themselves.
- The process of creativity is not dependent on conventional language or communication.
- The creative experience is usually followed by discussion, where feelings and thoughts are put into words.
- The product of the creative process can be used as a medium

for communication between members of the group.

- The group discussion encourages questions and comments which may help group members to gain a further understanding of their problems and their emotional responses.
- The creative session provides space, time, safety and permission for spontaneous expression.
- Participants are 'allowed' to have fun, to play, to explore and experiment in ways rarely permitted to adults.

Although many creative techniques are employed in occupational therapy, not all are appropriate to creative therapy. Any that demand specific technical skill, such as engraving; any that involve the use of complex machinery, such as printing; or any that are particularly slow, such as wood carving, would not normally be classified as creative therapies. The activity must provide a means of spontaneously experiencing, exploring and communicating emotion and then provide a medium for verbal communication. Participation in the activity encourages dyadic or group interaction, and offers opportunities for participants to experiment with self-disclosure.

Creative therapies are often carried out in groups. There are potential benefits for participants to see problems which mirror their own, and hear these discussed by a group. The actions of the group in creative therapies may have a condensing effect, so that the 'collective energy of the group...may intensify feelings' (Stockwell 1988). It is the process, not the product of the creative session, which is of primary importance, although the product may provide the focus for discussion and future action. Also, as Foulkes (1984) said, 'it is the process of communication rather than the content of the information it conveys which is important to us'.

Creative therapies generally share a similar organisation. The session divides into an experiential period followed by a time for discussion. Often the activity is undertaken with a group, who may be selected for a closed group, or participants may have more flexible membership in open groups. The activity takes place for a predetermined period of time and ideally occurs in a quiet area where interruptions are avoided. There is usually an expectation that all group members will participate, although clients who are reluctant or anxious may observe initial sessions. Non-participant observers, particularly staff who do not share the experiential work but expect to contribute to the discussion period, are not usually encouraged.

The roles and relationships within a creative therapy group are based on democratic principles, or at least on those of a guided democracy. Each member is equally respected, has equal rights to contribute, and no opinion is considered more valuable than another. Each has the right to determine his or her own level of involvement, the amount of self-disclosure during discussion and to have control over any creative work produced. It is often the case that the experience of staff, their involvement in the planning and management of the session and their paid position within the hospital may alter role perceptions and group dynamics.

MODELS OF PRACTICE
Psychological models

Creative therapies have emerged from humanist and psychoanalytic models, but they contain within them many eclectic philosophies drawn from psychology, rehabilitation and occupational therapy. Each therapy and each therapist may base practice on different blends of theory, and there may be considerable disagreement about their source. What follows is a review of creative therapy practice and the models which have been influential to its development and use.

Psychoanalysis

The analytical schools of psychiatry have been most influential in the development of psychodrama and analytical art therapy. The main elements which characterise this model are that:

- The patient's difficulties arise from early childhood experiences which are reflected in problems in adult relationships.
- Emotional conflicts often remain unresolved through the persistent use of defence mechanisms, but the person remains unaware of the source of these difficulties.
- Interpretation of creative actions or products by the therapist will help the person to gain insight.
- Creative therapy offers an alternative route to the unconscious through the interpretation of symbols.
- Creative therapy encourages a realisation that defence mechanisms are used persistently in a variety of situations and that patterns of reactions can be discerned throughout life.

- Therapy aims to help people gain insight into the source and nature of conflicts within their life, and this knowledge can provide them with basic information on how and why they might change.
- Therapy offers safe environments where emotions can be explored and expressed, so catharsis can encourage insight and vice versa.
- Group therapy recognises that many people share inadequate and unsuccessful patterns of behaviour.
- Group discussion following the creative activity can promote insight, catharsis and problem solving.

This approach requires the clients actively to 'show' the therapist and the group their interpersonal and emotional conflicts, rather than to 'tell' them. In drama therapy, for example, a protagonist, or central 'player' volunteers or emerges from the group during the warm-up discussion phase of the group. The therapist/director and the rest of the group assist this person to enact situations through which the conflict may become understood. The therapist is responsible for setting the stage, directing the action and helping the protagonist to select and use the other group members in their roles of auxiliary egos or doubles. The director also suggests changes and developments to the action, involving different techniques such as role reversal, mirroring, aggressive release or talking to an empty chair. An essential responsibility for the therapist is the closure of the group, where protagonists and auxiliary egos are de-roled.

Projective art work also is linked to analytic theory. The art work is seen as a projection of unconscious defence mechanisms and unresolved psychological conflicts. The symbolism within the work becomes the therapist's focus, where particular imagery, use of colour or spatial relationships are considered to have particular meaning. Assael & Popovici-Wacks (1989) state: 'the symbols are much more expressive and relevant to the mental state of the patient, because he chooses his specific symbols for his specific condition.' In projective art, patients free-associate through the painting or modelling as part of the analytic process. In these art and drama groups, the therapist, trained in analysis, interprets the work of the group, although in many situations the group are also encouraged to contribute to the interpretation.

Humanist and Gestalt therapy

The humanist, existential and Gestalt schools have had considerable impact on the development of drama therapy, encounter groups and the use of art activities which are generally termed creative therapies. These therapies draw from Rogers and Perls and have the common elements that:

- Each individual is seen as being unique, rational and constructive and capable of moving forward to self-directed goals.
- The clients have the ability to understand and solve their own problems.
- Therapy sessions permit the experience of personal responsibility and exploration of previously denied attitudes.
- The conflicts and problems which are most important to the client will probably emerge first.
- The therapist is non-judgemental, attempts to empathise fully with the client and maintains at all times an empathetic and non-judgemental approach to each individual.
- The creative activity and subsequent shared discussion, help all group members to gain an understanding of how other members perceive their lives; their own 'universe of one' (Schon 1982).

In remedial drama the group comes together and discusses individual or group conflicts. The therapist, or experienced group members, may suggest 'games' which will assist people to explore these further. If the group is aware that communication is a problem, a number of nonverbal activities, chanting or word games may be suggested. The therapist often participates in these games, and may take responsibility for their organisation and timing. The group come together to discuss their perceptions of the group's actions and debate the different meanings they may have had for each individual. The therapist does not impose her view on the others, but encourages the group to clarify meanings. Similarly, in art groups, the work and the group dynamics of the session are interpreted by the participants.

Behaviourism

Behaviourism has been influential in the development of sociodrama. The aim of these groups is to role play social roles and tasks. The participants are rewarded for approximation in their role play to that of the therapist's model. Rewards of praise or points are given by the therapist as new social skills are learned and successfully practised. There is a distinct difference in approach between sociodrama and the drama techniques employed in creative therapy. Sociodrama is not considered to be a creative therapy, because it is concerned with behavioural products, not the process of self-discovery.

Aspects of behaviourism are inherent in all social situations, including creative therapy groups. The approval of the therapist and the group for attendance, participation and conformity to group norms provide reinforcement to each group member. The extent to which the therapist manipulates this effect will influence the dynamics of the group and the eventual outcomes.

The application of the psychological models

To emphasise how psychological models influence both the action and interpretation of creative work, I will focus on four specific aspects of therapy:

- spontaneous expression
- self-exploration in a safe environment
- communicating emotion to oneself and others
- active involvement in therapy.

All creative therapies emphasise the importance of spontaneous expression. Davies (1987) suggests that we neglect 'our creativity, spontaneity, drama, horror, playfulness, ritual, dance, body movement, physical contact, fantasy, music and nonverbal communication'. So each technique aims to diminish the barriers which may interrupt free expression. Warm-up exercises, full group involvement, excluding observers, and offering secluded locations can decrease embarrassment and social inhibition. Psychoanalytical models associate spontaneous expression with free association, which allows the individual to make and see new connections between thoughts and experiences and thereby gain insight into his or her personality. In analytical models of creative work, such as psychodrama, the therapist makes these analyses from his observations of the clients and by interpreting the symbolism of their work. The interpretations are related to the clients' past life experiences.

Humanist models perceive spontaneous expression as a means of overcoming what Rogers (1974) describes as 'an unwillingness to communicate self' and a 'tendency to only communicate about external events'. The 'I and Thou, Here-and-Now' (Perls 1973) of Gestalt therapy is central to the therapeutic process, focusing on the unique perceptions and cognition of each person, and the central importance of present experiences. Creative works or actions have no intrinsic meaning relating to the past, in this model. Only the individual client can impart meaning to it, and that meaning may change over time. Through discussion of actions which are not planned or rehearsed in advance, the person is helped to become aware of 'how he is producing his difficulties, he can see what his present difficulties are, and he can solve them in the present' (Perls 1973).

Spontaneous expression must occur in a 'safe' environment. Within the psychoanalytic model, safety is created by having closed membership and consistent, trustworthy leadership by the analyst/therapist. In the humanist model, safety is created by the trust which develops within the group, and through the unconditional positive regard of therapist for clients, and group members for each other. It is a dilemma whether the safety created by assisting people to participate provides the best condition in which spontaneous expression and self-discovery can occur. Goodman suggests that the 'very worst thing you can do for people is to help them' (Glascow 1971) and that frustrating demands for support and help will help clients to discover their own capabilities and potential for problem solving. Perls (1969) suggested that the goal of therapy is the client's realisation that 'what he expects from the therapist, he can do just as well himself'. So, while providing sufficient safety for participation, the therapist does not deny the client a place to take and experience risk.

There are different views about the nature and source of the emotional expression through creativity. In psychoanalysis the expression is thought to arise through catharsis. Freud adopted the term 'catharsis' to describe the feeling of relief following a period of tension or psychological conflict. The intensity of these emotions may be surprising to both the client and the therapist but may 'purge the unconscious of troublesome repressed material and provide an increase in insight' (Thompson & Mathias 1994). Erikson (1968) believed that emotions arose from unresolved conflicts at different stages of life. Humanists see emotions, such as frustration or anger, accompanying an impasse to self-actualisation; elation might occur when these barriers are successfully overcome.

Creative therapies encourage the individual to experiment with new forms of action and emotional reaction to events. Creative therapies may be equivalent to play, and facilitate people's natural tendency to learn and develop through fantasy and social and constructive play, which are often denied to adults. People can play at being emotional. Emotions to play situations may be transient and part of the play activity itself, so that the person can experiment with feeling elated or sad.

The process of personal change is also explained differently by each model. The analytic approach sees change occurring through insight. Creative activities expose elements of the unconscious, which, when explained to the client, will 'redirect psychic energy to the rational goal-choosing ego' (Young & Quinn 1992). The humanists see the change occurring as part of motivation towards self-actualisation. Developmental models suggest that, just as the child passes through stages of development, often in sequential orders, the damaged body and mind may repeat some aspects of these developmental sequences during recovery. In psychiatric illness social withdrawal is common, and creative therapy may encourage people to move from solitary, to associative, then parallel, and finally cooperative interactions with others. Mosey (1989) stresses the importance of 'recapitulation' to the psychiatric patient, and creative therapies can offer opportunities for patients to revisit and work out problems of psychosocial development.

Creative therapies are action therapies. Their use as an analytical technique is distinctly different from the usual passive talking approach. Moreno's development of psychodrama created a completely new form of analysis, where the individual was required to act-out life conflicts and dilemmas. Both psychoanalytic and humanist theories in creative therapy stress the importance of using action to bypass the barriers which occur in spoken communication. The techniques encourage and permit physical expression, physical contact and access to thoughts and emotion through nonverbal channels.

There are inevitable differences of opinion among practising therapists about the rationale underpinning their individual work. There are clear cases where specific models predominate: psychoanalytic theories in psychodrama; Gestalt theory in encounter groups; behaviourism in sociodrama. But even here there will be disagreements and differences in interpretation. The situation is made confused by the inconsistency with which terms are applied to techniques. The terms 'drama therapy', 'art therapy' and 'music therapy' may be applied to many different techniques, which emphasise different staff roles and responsibilities and goals.

Rehabilitation models

Creative therapy plays an important role in the 'needs' and 'roles' models (Ekdawi & Conning 1994) of psychiatric rehabilitation. Creative therapies are concerned with helping people to identify their needs and the barriers which thwart self-discovery and achievement. Regrettably, current practice emphasises the role of staff in gathering information about clients, to identify their needs and then construct a relevant treatment programme. In creative therapy, the clients present their perceptions of their life and identify their own needs. Reviewing the literature, Ekdawi & Conning suggest that the word 'need', has become interchangeable for staff with 'problem', 'demand', 'want', 'resources offered by a professional', or 'a standard defined by a professional'. Creative therapies place no stress on acquiring skills or meeting health professionals' needs. What they offer is an opportunity for clients to explore their own goals and discuss these with others. Knowledge and skill are acquired through self-discovery learning.

The role model of rehabilitation has some relevance to creative therapy. Creative activity functions at a number of levels. It offers opportunities for participants to examine the roles they hold in society, some of which may be reflected in the roles they choose to hold within the group. Creative therapy sessions aim to challenge traditional staff/patient/sick roles, by requiring active involvement and valuing individual contributions. Group members are challenged to review their responses to illness and roles which they have adopted in relation to them. The sessions will inevitably challenge the traditional roles held by medical and therapy staff.

Occupational therapy models

The aims of creative therapy link closely with the object relations goals of OT defined by Bruce & Borg (1987) by offering a route for emotional expression, a means to improve ego functioning, a technique to establish self-control, and a way to learn and test out new skills and roles. The developmental models proposed by Fidler (Fidler & Fidler 1963) and Mosey (1989) have some relevance, but more in terms of group interaction than through the therapy itself. However, there has been increasing emphasis on the human occupation model of therapy within the last decade, which is more concerned with skill acquisition than the emotional and spiritual development and well-being of the client.

Creative therapies offer a very particular opportunity for clients. There is no specific need for assessment prior to participation, although some therapists may have criteria for exclusion from the group. The client's assessment of his problems, dysfunction and environmental difficulties is shared with the therapist and the group, and is achieved through the individual's interpretation of his work and his experience of the group. The therapist facilitates group interaction through session preparation, but often achieves most when doing least, by allowing the group to be self-directing and motivating. The activity offers opportunities for continuous self-evaluation by the client through reflection and discussion.

Creative therapists—specialists or generalists?

There has been considerable controversy about who should be responsible for creative therapies. There are now a significant number of courses offering qualifications in art, drama, dance/ movement and music therapy with participants in these courses coming from both art and therapy backgrounds. Creative therapies are taught in undergraduate and postgraduate occupational therapy courses.

The skills of the specialist art therapists offer a significant contribution to the treatment and rehabilitation of clients with psychiatric problems. Their expertise with a medium is exciting and motivating to group participants, and their greater experience with a single treatment modality offers particular understandings of the therapy. Many specialist creative therapists complain of professional stereotyping which focuses on the artistic product, rather than the process, and of confusions between art workshops and creative therapy. The old spectre of diversionary activity comes back to haunt both occupational and specialist therapists.

Since the inception of specialist courses, there has been controversy about what relationships should evolve between each of these specialist therapies, and between them and occupational therapy. In many units, the specialist therapists share occupational therapy department space and, in most of these, multidisciplinary work practices have developed. However, there have been fears that specialist therapists have taken over areas which were traditionally part of occupational therapy, leading to role confusion and fragmented responsibility. Occupational therapists use creative therapies as part of an integrated, holistic programme of treatment which is concerned with all aspects of life skills and spiritual and emotional well-being. Clearly, the expectation that specialist therapists should be subordinate to occupational therapists is inappropriate, but the various professional groups and individual teams need to define how treatment programmes, assessments and evaluations can be coordinated, and therapy offered in coherent and meaningful ways to clients. This will be particularly important in the context of purchaser/provider markets.

Both occupational therapists and specialist therapists need in turn to review their relationship to the 'talking' therapists of psychoanalysis and counselling. There has traditionally been a view that, while creative work offered alternative media for communication, the data it generated should be examined during individual or small closed psychotherapy groups. Therapists need to consider how creativity can be both therapeutic activity in its own right and an adjunct to psychotherapy. Excessive splintering of therapeutic effort can be confusing for both clients and therapists and lead to fragmented understanding of problems and uncoordinated focuses of problem solving.

THE THERAPEUTIC PROCESS

This section does not attempt to offer instruction about the content of creative therapy sessions, but highlights the particular problems of client selection, leadership, group initiation and closure, and evaluation, when these therapies are being used as part of an occupational therapy programme.

Client selection

There have always been disagreements about the suitability of certain diagnostic groups for creative therapy sessions. The view that only the young, verbally able, intelligent and sensitive clients could benefit from analysis, has spilled over into discussions about creative therapies. There are suggestions that those experiencing psychotic symptoms are unable to participate because of lack of insight and loss of contact with reality; that the depressed are unable to express emotion; that the old reject the activity as being childish; and that the agitated, aggressive or regressed patients are unsuitable because of their inability to contribute to group work and discussion. This leaves the therapist with a singularly small group with whom to work.

There are, however, many accounts of creative therapies being used with just such groups. Assael and Popovici-Wacks (1989) suggest that it is a false belief that depressed patients are not creative, for while verbal communication may be suppressed 'it is much easier to paint than talk and write' and they are 'able to overcome the inhibition of depression, guilt feelings, self accusations and self depreciation'.

Huddleston (1989) describes the value of drama therapy with the elderly to 'promote group cohesion and development, together with personal growth' while Drucker (1990) has outlined the value of creative experience to the well-being of elderly clients in her health district. Diagnostic classification is not a particularly useful guideline for predicting who might benefit from creative therapy. Florid psychotic symptoms, gross agitation or the threat of self- or group-harm are usually seen as temporary bars to group participation, but the activities may still be used on an individual basis with considerable therapeutic effect.

Creative therapists would generally agree that clients should not be compelled or coerced into participation. The same is true of students and junior staff, whose obligatory presence in a group can have negative effects on the group, especially when their involvement is transitory. Each therapist has to reflect on how clients can be best encouraged to participate, through giving information, offering support, or allowing passive observation before making a commitment, and what the implications will be for the client and the dynamics of the group.

There are controversies about if and how clients should be selected for groups, the merits of open or closed groups, or whether groups should have mixed or single diagnoses, symptoms or problems. Individual therapists will have their own view based on the philosophy of their practice and the traditions and experience of their unit.

Group leadership

It has already been suggested that therapists do not participate as 'leaders' in creative therapy sessions. Descriptors such as facilitator or enabler are often used to avoid the implication that the therapist has control over group actions. Those with special analytical training may acquire the role of expert leader, but therapists usually attempt to establish more equitable roles with the clients.

What the therapist offers to the group is:

- Acceptance and empathy, which may be absent in the clients' family, work or social life.
- A willingness to be involved in the content and emotion of the clients' lives. The therapist attempts to understand beliefs from the clients' perspectives, not from the therapist's view point.
- Opportunities for therapeutic relationships to mirror or model relationships which may occur outside the group. In analytical terms there may be transference between client and therapist.
- Jargon-free explanations of what might be happening within the dynamics of the group and judgement-free comments about creative work.
- Honest reflection about his or her personal experiences and emotions in the group which might influence interactions. These may be shared with the group or may be used by the therapist with a mentor in supervision sessions. The recognition of bias towards certain individuals or behaviours is seen as crucial to effective group work.
- Minimal direction but optimal encouragement and empowerment throughout the creative session.

The predominantly Rogerian principles outlined here are not always easy to implement. For the therapist, it is 'no longer important to make the "right" interpretations, but instead to offer suggestions, provide alternatives, ways of looking at things, to challenge assumptions and generally to attempt to provide a very active feedback and response' (Connell & Wright 1994). Yet therapists may have autocratic leadership roles thrust upon them, by the expectation of either other staff or clients. When challenging behaviour occurs within the group, the therapist is expected to take responsibility for group safety. Many therapists find that their inclination to help leads them to advise, instruct and inform in a way that is out of kilter with humanist creative therapy principles. The experienced therapist learns to 'tolerate uncertainty and chaos' (McNeilly 1990) without immediately imposing his own organisation and structure on the group. Bruce & Borg (1987) suggest that 'the therapist who is most comfortable with herself, able to communicate concern and able to see her own responsibilities, is most able to foster a helping relationship and movement in therapy'. Such abilities develop through experience and active reflective practice.

The possible roles which a therapist may be expected to hold as leader are facilitator, expert, boss, adviser or controller. Such multiplicity of roles can be confusing and demanding. It is common practice for some responsibilities to be shared with a co-therapist, who shares the workload of preparation and offers alternative views in group feedback. The co-therapist can observe the group when the therapist may be offering information to the group or guiding discussion. He can also diffuse the perception of the therapist as an 'expert' or 'boss' by questioning or challenging her in the group, and so provide a role model for group members to do the same. In times of crisis, the therapists are able to maintain the group even if one is dealing with interruptions or disturbances. Finlay (1993) describes the advantages of co-therapy as mutual support and the development of each other's professional skills through reflection and discussion. Disadvantages only arise if the therapists do not share common goals, theoretical orientations or attitudes to leadership.

Leadership roles may evolve during the life of the group. There may be a period where the therapist needs to counteract the fears and unrealistic expectations clients might have about creative work, by taking control of aspects of the group before encouraging the gradual development of assertiveness and responsibility by all group members. The danger may be, that having established power and control relationships, these are difficult to renounce at a later stage. The old adage, 'To lead people, walk behind them', is a guiding principle in creative work.

Therapists may face a number of personal and professional dilemmas when establishing their role within the group. Offering personal information about their own work establishes equity in the group, but they may find the fine line between participation and using the group as their own therapy a difficult one to tread. Co-therapists, especially if joined by a cohort of other staff, may appear to clients less as participants than as an imposing and opposing force of experts. For many therapists, allowing group members to take full responsibility for themselves, to control the group and to determine its actions runs contrary to their normal roles. The tendency to advise and control is difficult to renounce. Bruce & Borg (1987) summarise the facilitative role as being a 'knowledgeable, empathetic guide who develops a collaborative relationship with the patient and maintains the framework of treatment.'

Initiation and closure

Like any good story, a creative therapy session needs a clear beginning and end. Whether the group is selected, open or closed, members need some explanation of the activity and the boundaries and expectations which apply. Some introductions and broad guidelines may need to be given. What plagues the therapist is that selection, encouragement to join groups, and scene setting and guidance can all reinforce his or her leadership of the group. There is a fine dividing line between excessive structuring leading to group dependence and passivity, and inadequate structuring which leads to anxiety, avoidance and frustration. Groups may vary in the amount of support they need to begin work and maintain their motivation.

However, no particular preparation can guarantee efficient group cooperation, and most groups will pass through periods of forming, norming and storming before there is efficient performing (Tuckman, 1965). The dynamics of every group are very different: some can become quickly exclusive; others remain open to new members. Some establish fixed roles for members; others allow roles to change or blurred responsibilities to occur. Some groups will quickly take personal and group responsibilities; others will always be fragmented and unproductive. The group need to continuously review the dynamics of their interactions, so that each session is a development from the last.

Members need to know when a group is going to end, so that people can prepare to leave a session or a programme. Final exercises incorporate aspects of social rituals of leaving so that participants do not leave with a sense of dissatisfaction making them overly excited or overtly upset. It would be unrealistic and inappropriate to expect that there will not be feelings of frustration, anger, happiness and a sense of unfinished business created by the group, but these are acknowledged so that any unfinished business is identified. Where sessions form part of a series or holistic treatment programme, these feelings become the material for subsequent groups. People should, it is hoped, leave the group with a sense that the costs of participation have not outweighed the benefits.

In psychiatry, growth and personal development may begin at the end of a treatment period, or even at some time distant to it. The therapist may need to consider a number of 'endings' to groups: those at the end of each session; the end of a series of sessions; and the closure which may come if the group finally meets for a follow-up discussion some time after the sessions have been completed. Evaluation of progress may be quite different on each of these occasions.

Assessment and evaluation

Creative therapies include personal and group evaluation within each session. All members of the group are encouraged to discuss interpersonal relationships within the group and often use these observations as material for subsequent sessions. Clients and staff in groups are encouraged to use reflection in and reflection on their actions within the group. Clients may also plan 'homework' in response to these reflections, to test out new insights, social or emotional responses between sessions, and thereby gain continuous assessment of their progress. Some therapists use the final session of a closed, fixed-term group to review past work and review changes which have occurred to individuals and the group. Some therapists employ pre- and post-therapy assessment questionnaires, which offer additional quantitative and qualitative evidence.

Therapists use debriefing techniques after each group, to share and clarify perceptions with the group and then with their multidisciplinary team. Many also find staff support groups, mentoring or supervision invaluable to reflect outside the group about how their personal attitudes might be influencing the group, as part of their professional development. In the absence of such support, reflective journals can provide the therapist with information about the dynamics of creative therapy sessions.

There is little research data available about the efficacy of creative therapies in occupational therapy. Crouch (1987) reported the value of art therapy for quick and efficient assessment of the client, and that such assessments had high interrelater reliability with other procedures used by other members of the multidisciplinary team. There is less evidence concerning the efficacy of specific techniques in treatment. Moreno (1968) stated that 'the validity of psychodrama does not require proof beyond its face value' for client reports and therapist observations served as validation. In contrast, Kane (1992) recommends that quantitative research should be increased and updated, focusing particularly on the suitability of techniques for specific client groups, and that trained therapists report their experiences more widely in journals and at conferences.

There are profound problems in measuring the effectiveness of creative therapies. They rarely exist as a single treatment modality, and positive outcomes are difficult to separate from other concurrent psychotherapies. Measuring patient participation and degree of cooperation in therapy could lead to the mistaken equation of treatment success with compliance or productivity. Client self-evaluation and reporting is coherent with the philosophy of the techniques, but the timing, anticipated audience, or desire to please the therapist need to be recognised as factors that may bias the findings.

Evaluation of the group by use of video recordings, sociograms, or event measurement can help the therapist and group to optimise their individual and group effort. Outcomes of such evaluations can be shared and used as topics for creative sessions. The aim, methodology and ethics of assessment all need to be carefully considered before such material can be released to audiences outside the group. But more research into creative therapy is urgently needed.

Problems and barriers

For many people, the experience of art, music and drama in school confirmed their opinion that it was something they could not do, being accessible only to a talented elite. The daily exposure to the arts provides a standard which they know they cannot equal. We know what a good picture should look like, or how good music should sound. Introducing creative therapy to clients, already low in self-esteem and confidence, is often met with antagonism or apathy.

The association of arts with school also creates a second barrier. Many people think of painting or pottery, drama or movement as essentially childish pursuits. Most adults are encouraged to put away childish things and take on adult responsibilities. Play is charged with being both time wasting and immoral. Involvement in it is both potentially embarrassing, irrelevant and demeaning. Where illness, diagnosis and treatment already emphasise dependence and adult inadequacy, the suggestion of regressing to childish pursuits may generate a real sense of worthlessness. For the artistically talented, the use of art in a context that devalues skill may equally result in resistance and rejection of the techniques.

The therapist has to ask whether reluctant clients should be confronted, encouraged or ignored. If the resistance is seen as a form of communication in its own right and part of the creative process, by engaging the therapist in a 'push–pull struggle' (Rusek 1991), the overcoming of reticence, the challenging of authority, or the determination not to participate, can be positive therapeutic outcomes. There will be complex reasons for non-participation, but these are an integral part of creative therapy, not preliminary or separate to it. There are likely to be problems throughout the life span of the group: rejection of aggressive or inadequate members by the group; monopoly of the group by dominant members; scapegoating; refusal to participate; silence; or running away or absenteeism. Creative therapists may encounter more problems because of the active nature of the sessions and their focus on group interactions.

The ownership of creative work, particularly in writing and painting can be problematic. The public display of work changes the creative purpose from being a means of gaining insight, expressing emotion and interacting with others, to a product-centred activity for an audience. Clients are free to destroy work at the end of sessions, or may choose to keep a personal portfolio for use in other psychotherapies, or for personal reflection. The therapist is often faced with deciding how and when to dispose of work, and whether it might have relevance to clients if they are readmitted.

Some barriers to participation are related to psychiatric symptoms, such as problems with verbal communication, withdrawal from interpersonal relationships, unconscious denial or projection of problems and loss of motivation. More covertly, both staff and patients may be reluctant to give up the advantages of their traditional staff/patient roles.

Futures

Serrett (1985) suggests that in the current trends in psychiatric care towards biological treatment and cost containment, therapy will become less concerned with self-expression and personal growth and more with activities related to occupational competency. The closure of psychiatric hospitals will also lead to a reduction of venues where therapies occur. Although day hospitals and units are being established, space and facilities are often limited. The social market view of psychiatric care has become prevalent, where the outcomes of treatment are 'construed as quantifiable products which can be clearly pre-specified in tangible and concrete form' (Elliott 1991).

Occupational therapists have a traditional grounding in medical science, are committed to tests and measurements, evaluation procedures and quality assurance measures. This science background has promoted a belief that the therapist is an expert able to use these measurement tools to judge the patient's problem and select a relevant therapy. This technical and rational approach encourages the notion that the therapist's evaluation is correct and can be imposed on the client. Questioning or refusal to accept this interpretation is seen as non-compliance with treatment. Despite therapists' espousal of humanist paradigms and holistic practice in psychiatry, pressure to conform to new business practices in medicine has placed a considerable obligation on therapists. Creative therapies are experiential, and the outcomes unpredictable and even unquantifiable in the short term. Such treatment methodologies, which emphasise emotional and spiritual effects, fit uneasily with managers seeking measurable behavioural outcomes. Creative work also encourages clients to gain emancipatory knowledge which reduces their dependence on expert wisdom to make them well. Where professionals are under threat, there is danger in supporting methodologies which appear to negate professionalism.

Yet perhaps the need for creative therapy is greater now than ever before. There is increasing disillusion with medicine and growing acceptance that individuals have a potential to change and meet their own goals. Where psychiatric intervention has produced limited benefits, many clients gain self-knowledge and experience human contact through creative work. Its retention as part of community psychiatric treatment may not be easy, but may offer an important tool to counteract the despair and isolation which so many people experience.

REFERENCES

Assael M, Popovici-Wacks M 1989 Artistic expression in spontaneous paintings of depressed patients. Israel Journal of Psychiatry Related Sciences 26(4): 223–243

Bruce M A, Borg B 1987 Frames of reference in psychosocial occupational therapy. Slack, New York

Busuttil J 1990 An art therapy exhibition: a retrospective view. British Journal of Occupational Therapy 53(12): 501–503

Connell C, Wright R 1994 Art therapy. In: Wells R, Tschudin V (eds) Wells' Supportive therapies in health care. Baillière Tindall, London

Crouch R B 1987 A study of the effectiveness of certain occupational therapy group techniques in the assessment of the acutely disturbed adult psychiatric patient. British Journal of Occupational Therapy 50(3): 86–90

Davies M H 1987 Dramatherapy and psychodrama. In: Jennings S (ed) Dramatherapy: theory and practice for teachers and clinicians. Croom Helm, London

Drucker K L 1990 Swimming upstream. In: Liebermann M (ed) Art therapy in practice. Jessica Kingsley Publishers, London

Ekdawi M Y, Conning A M 1994 Psychiatric rehabilitation: a practical guide. Chapman & Hall, London

Elliott J 1991 Three perspectives on coherence and continuity in teacher education. Paper prepared for UCET Annual Conference, Nov 1991

Erikson E H 1968 Identity: youth and crisis. Norton, New York

Fidler G S, Fidler J W 1963 Occupational therapy: a communication process in psychiatry. Macmillan, New York

Finlay L 1993 Groupwork in occupational therapy. Therapy in practice No. 38. Chapman & Hall, London

Foulkes S H 1984 Therapeutic group analysis. Allyn & Unwin, London

Glascow R 1971 Paul Goodman: a conversation. Psychology Today (Nov): 62–96

Huddleston R 1989 Drama with elderly people. British Journal of Occupational Therapy 52(8): 298–300

Kane R 1992 The potential abuses, limitations and negative effects of classical psychodramatic techniques in group counseling. Journal of Group Psychotherapy, Psychodrama and Sociometry 4(4): 181–189

Kirschenbaum H, Henderson V L (eds) 1989 The Carl Rogers reader. Constable, London

McNeilly G 1990 Group analysis and art therapy: a personal perspective. Group Analysis 23(3): 215–224

Moreno J L 1968 The validity of psychodrama groups. Psychotherapy 21: 3

Mosey A C 1989 Recapitulation of ontogenesis: a theory for the practice of occupational therapy. American Journal of Occupational Therapy 22: 426–438

Parten M 1932 Social participation among pre-school children. Journal of Abnormal and Social Psychology 12: 243–269. Cited in: Berk L 1991 Child development, 2nd edn. Allyn & Bacon, Boston

Perls F S 1969 Gestalt therapy verbatim. Real People Press, Lafayette CA

Perls F S 1973 The Gestalt approach and eye witness to therapy. Bantam Books, New York

Rogers C R 1974 On becoming a person. Constable, London

Rusek J 1991 A creative approach to the treatment of resistance. Creative Therapy Review 12: 9–15

Schon D A 1982 The reflective practitioner: how professionals think in action. Basic Books, New York

Serrett K D 1985 Another look at occupational therapy's history: paradigm or pair-of-hands. In: Serrett K D (ed) 1985 Philosophical and historical roots of occupational therapy. Haworth Press, New York

Stockwell R 1988 Creative therapies. In: Willson M (ed) Occupational therapy in short-term psychiatry, 2nd edn. Churchill Livingstone, Edinburgh

Thompson T, Mathias T (eds) Lyttle's Mental health and disorder, 2nd edn. Baillière Tindall, London

Tuckman B W 1965 Developmental sequence in small groups. Psychology Bulletin 63: 384–399. Cited in: Argyle M 1969 Social interaction. Methuen, London

Young M E, Quinn E 1992 Theories and principles of occupational therapy. Churchill Livingstone, Edinburgh

10

Leisure

Christine Ravetz

AN EXPLORATION AND APPLICATION

This chapter will explore the concept of leisure, addressing relevant variables such as time, state of mind, work, gender, family, age, class, education, money, industry, cultural background and choice which affect leisure patterns. It will explore physical and psychosocial issues which affect participation in leisure activities. Finally, it will apply this knowledge to occupational therapy practice.

Definition. Leisure is time when a person involves him- or herself in activity, or non-activity, of his or her free will, for pleasure not remuneration, and enjoys a feeling of well-being, relaxation or stimulation.

The core notions in leisure are time and a feeling of well-being but there are also other influential variables.

VARIABLES WHICH AFFECT LEISURE PATTERNS
Time

Time is a fundamental consideration as it entails temporal space to be used, in this case, for some form of satisfying and chosen involvement. People have always had time set aside for special occasions such as: religious festivals like Christmas, Chanukah, Little Bairam or Dewali which invoke positive and joyous communion; family celebrations, for example weddings, which recognise rites of passage; and community celebrations such as harvest time which are congratulatory and socially binding. Such occasions provide a continuity to the notion of leisure because they all invoke a familiar feeling of individual, family or societal well-being.

Leisure as an important element of western society, however, has become more dominant during this century because of increased work-free time resulting from shorter working hours, underemployment, unemployment or use of labour-saving devices. These changes have resulted in more time being available for non-essential activities. In Britain, on average per week, men employed in paid work have 46 hours of leisure time, women in paid work have 31 hours, housewives have 52 hours, retired men have 90 hours and retired women have 70 hours (Social Trends 1994).

Leisure participation needs time. Time in itself, however, does not necessarily invoke leisure. Many people with time, such as the mentally ill, physically pained or psychosocially distressed, do not automatically experience pleasure. Many occupational therapy clients have time but are troubled.

State of mind

An essential element of leisure is a pleasurable state of mind. Leisure is a pleasant and chosen experience. It is not necessarily a free state as many pastimes involve commitment and restraint, for example playing for a sports team or child-centred activity. A positive state of mind is essential to leisure, although not exclusive to it. Many work-related activities can also produce such a state.

Work

The link between work and leisure is strong. The strongest links are:

- temporal in that leisure time is time left over from essential work activity—essential work activity may be waged when work involves production outside the domestic environment, or unwaged involving work necessary for personal or family well-being, such as domestic or care work
- financial in that waged work often provides the money to pay for leisure pursuits
- relational in that work interests and leisure interests may be strongly associated.

Parker (1976) contends that there are three distinct relationships between work and leisure which are:

- an extension pattern where work and leisure activities are blurred and are difficult to separate, for example playing golf with colleagues to undertake business may produce conflated work/leisure interests
- an opposition pattern where work and leisure activities are deliberately kept separate from each other, for example working in a hard, arduous industry and supporting the local football team on a Saturday afternoon
- a neutrality pattern when work and leisure are neither conflated nor kept apart, for example working in an office and dining out with work colleagues at the weekend solely because they are your friends.

Parker's last pattern also indicates another strong link between work and leisure, which is that many social contacts are made through work which extend and enrich leisure experiences. Grint (1991) also links work and leisure and tentatively offers the notion that 'in some sense work is the opposite of leisure'.

The link between work and leisure is not indisputable, however. One of the earliest works on leisure Veblen's *The Theory of the Leisure Class*, published in 1899, expounded that the rich, with plenty of leisure, held work and practical activity in contempt.

Gender

There are differences in leisure pursuits which relate to gender. Women's leisure tends to focus in or on the home. Men similarly focus on home-based activities such as do-it-yourself, but will also spend more time outside the home on sporting activities (passive or active), going to the pub or belonging to an organisation

(Green et al 1995). The withdrawal from sporting activities by young women tends to occur during adolescence. Difference in leisure patterns, however, manifests itself earlier than adolescence. More girls will attend dancing classes and ride horses and more boys will play football and play computer games, for example.

There are shared leisure activities, however, such as watching television, eating out, dancing, listening to music and visiting friends (General Household Survey 1983).

The family

In spite of gender differences in leisure habits, much leisure takes place within the family and involves commitment to mutually agreed activities which provide constraint and security as well as potential enjoyment, such as family holidays, educational visits and time spent together at festivals and celebrations. Kelly (1995) claims that people prefer the kind of leisure that is built upon intimate social relationships and place less value on total freedom. They experience 'role comfort' in an environment where they are known and accepted.

Age

Giddens (1993) divides the life cycle into five stages, which are childhood, adolescence, the young adult, mature adulthood and old age. His demarcation of the five stages will be used as a base from which to discuss leisure and age.

Childhood. In western society, childhood is recognised as special and is protected by the law. Unlike in former ages, children do not work full time in paid employment. For most, leisure time takes the form of play or time spent with people they know and trust such as family, friends or teachers and is oriented towards pleasure, development and learning. It can involve much contact with adults, although as children get older their relationships focus more and more on their peers, particularly of the same sex.

Adolescence. As in other areas of life, adolescents are in a transient stage between childhood and adulthood. Leisure pursuits are focused less on, or within, the family and more on peers of both sexes. Physical activity in the form of sports or dancing and self-identification (but within the constraints of peer group conformity and new experiences) dominate leisure choices.

The young adult. Educationally related ventures, politics, sexual experiences, travel and work concerns are likely to dominate young adult leisure. Later, activities which focus on interpersonal relationships and early family life become more prevalent.

Mature adulthood. Family-related or consumer-related leisure patterns may emerge. People may also plan for the future because of an expectation (not available to past generations) that life will be extended into old age.

Old age. Optimistically, old people can engage in renewal, particularly if finances are adequate and secure. New roles may be adopted, such as great-grandparenting, and work-free time may allow new skills to be learned. The less positive perspective implies financial insecurity, disengagement, loosened family ties and family disintegration, which will have negative effects on leisure. For all older people, more time is spent on activities of daily living such as washing, dressing, cleaning the home and shopping because these tasks take longer to do.

Some elderly are disadvantaged by low incomes but others, particularly the young elderly, have high incomes and are a target for the leisure industry as the growing number of holidays for the elderly indicates (Bond et al 1993).

Class and education

Several measures of social classification exist, the most well known probably being the Registrar General's Classification. Another more recently developed set of groupings is the Government Statistical Service Standard Occupational Classification (SOC). Both make a very strong link between occupation and class status and the latter, in particular, links social groupings with educational levels (Bond & Bond 1994). As the occupations at the top of both of these classifications involve long professional training, the link between class position and higher education is easy to make. Class position, education and higher income levels usually coincide. This relationship has implications for leisure activity. The situation is compounded by the very unequal distribution of wealth. According to Giddens (1993), 'The top 20% of households in 1991 received half of the total income for the population'. Poorer people will spend a greater proportion of their income on necessities such as food, fuel and light, clothing and transport. Consequently they will have proportionately less left over to spend on nonessentials like consumer leisure activities. They are also less likely to belong to clubs and societies or belong to organisations such as School Governors or The National Trust.

Money and industry

Leisure patterns are affected by the general economic state of both the country and the individual. Early industrialisation and urbanisation broke up or fundamentally modified pastimes relating to rural living and agriculture, such as harvest celebrations, sheep shearing and midsummer festivities (Hardy 1874). Cheap labour and the demands of industry dictated work patterns based on long working days and unpaid holidays. Changes in work practices, labour laws, unions and growth of new industries resulted in further mechanisation, shorter working weeks and paid holidays. The effect was more leisure time and higher wages. Contemporary work practices have produced a waged labour market for some and, for others, a flexible, less secure work career, unemployment or underemployment.

Linked to these changes is the growth of the leisure industry which targets the leisured person as consumer of related products. Leisure goods include caravans, music systems, sports goods, computer games, books and televisions. Leisure services include the theatre, holidays, eating out and theme parks. The enjoyment of these leisure products requires income in excess of that required for essential goods. As noted above, those on higher incomes will have more money to spend on these commodities. A lot of money is spent, however. In 1992 in the United Kingdom 17% of the household budget, on average, was spent on leisure (Social Trends 1994).

Cultural background

Culture is the social guidelines, rules, beliefs, norms and customs acquired by a member of society which affect that member's thinking and behaviour (Giddens 1993). People's leisure pursuits will be influenced by the culture into which they have been socialised.

Although not as varied as the United State of America, Britain is a heterogeneous nation whose citizens enjoy a plethora of historical, social and creative backgrounds. Knowledge of appropriate cultural differences will add to the therapeutic repertoire of an occupational therapist involved in leisure rehabilitation or management. Many customs appear to be universal, such as family gatherings, sharing food, talking, dancing and enjoying music. The method of their enactment, however, may be very different.

Enjoyment and appreciation of other people's culture also produces additional leisure interest.

Choice

⌐ne of the tenets of the concepts of leisure is choice. People ⌐ulge in activities of their own free will. The nature of leisure is ⌐eatened if coercion to participate occurs. Leisure time is time ⌐lled in chosen activity or non-activity. There are many kinds of leisure pursuits to choose from and some of them will be discussed in the next section.

DIFFERENT KINDS OF LEISURE ACTIVITIES

Types of leisure activity are not clearly differentiated and merge into each other:

- privatised leisure tends to occur within the family or home environment
- intimate groups of people like the family tend to go on holiday or on trips with each other
- holidays are highly commercialised as are other forms of leisure be they of a passive or active nature.

All of these categories of leisure pursuits offer a different perspective on the subject, however, and illustrate how rich the leisure world can be.

Privatised leisure

Privatised leisure involves the pursuit of activities in the privacy of the home. Roberts (1995) relates the increase in home-centredness to a highly mobile population, the demise of local communities and the strength of the nuclear family. It may also be due to increased comfort within the home provided by central heating, less overcrowding and the accumulation of affordable goods such as fitted carpets, comfortable furniture and home entertainment equipment such as televisions, music centres and video machines. Warmth, comfort and the availability of personal entertainment have possibly made staying in a very desirable leisure option. It must be remembered, however, that for many people, particularly women, the home has always been a central focus for other than work activities.

Watching television and videos and listening to the radio or music are some of the most popular activities undertaken by both sexes within the home. These activities appear to cut across all age and gender demarcations and are universally enjoyed within Britain. A fast-growing form of privatised leisure is playing computer games.

Do-it-yourself is another very popular home-based activity. This pursuit, if successful, saves money, creates a personalised living space which in appearance is part of self-image and self-presentation, adds further to the comfort of staying at home and, consequently, may increase privatisation. The do-it-yourself ideal may be better than the reality but, nevertheless, it is appealing and entices people, particularly men, to spend money and time on this type of occupation.

Cooking is very popular, as the plethora of cooking programmes on the television and the large amount of cookery books and kitchen equipment which are sold and bought indicate. Perusal of a mainstream supermarket bookshelf, let alone a speciality book shop, indicates the wide range of easy ways to produce meals and methods of cooking which are available to suit different tastes and pockets.

Family leisure

Closely linked with privatised leisure is family leisure which, as is mentioned above, offers security, constraints, commitment and anticipated, and often fulfilled, enjoyment. Pursuits range from family holidays, of which there are an infinite variety, to watching television together. It certainly involves communal meals and the celebration of festivals and special family events. In spite of the stresses relating to family life, it is very popular and well catered for by the service industries.

Holidays

Clarke & Critcher (1995) describe the holiday as a 'lived fantasy' which dominates the whole year. Holidays involve decisions, planning, preparation and anticipation of an extended period of pleasurable time. Almost 60% of the British population take at least one holiday per year, some taking two or three. The most popular British holiday locations are the West Country, Scotland and Wales. An increasing number of people take holidays abroad, with a growing number going to the United States of America and Portugal. The seaside remains a popular destination (Social Trends 1994).

The wide variety of holidays available cater for all tastes, ranging from quiet, reflective solitary holidays to those which focus on specific age groups or interests such as holidays for the elderly, the 18 to 30 age range and sports or family holidays.

Akin to holidays requiring sleeping away from home, are short trips to visit selected locations or events such as horse racing and the Boat Show; areas of scenic beauty; sporting occasions and theme parks.

Commercial leisure

People spend money on leisure, and both the private and public sectors are major providers, catering for growing demand and often making large profits from leisure spending. The link with work is also strong because the leisure industry creates jobs. There are industries which make goods such a sports shoes, clothes and equipment which aim beyond the functional and link with the highly successful fashion industry to provide goods which develop self-presentation. Products such as high tech tennis rackets or wine-making equipment assist the improvement of expertise and skills. Other industries such as leisure parks provide the activity direct, the two most popular in Britain being Blackpool Pleasure Beach (which draws international visitors) and Alton Towers. Other leisure parks, such as Disney World in Florida, Williamsburg in Virginia or Styal Mill in Greater Manchester, offer day trips or focused holidays that relate to a theme based on entertainment or historical interest. Theme parks relate to the 'lived fantasy' and have a 'feel good' factor necessary for a pleasurable state of mind. They are diverting and interesting and can be educational.

Mass entertainment also provides diversion and edification, examples being the cinema (cinema attendance has increased among the young since the introduction of multiplexes), the theatre with musicals being the most popular form, and major sports events such as Wimbledon and football finals which play to sell-out crowds and in addition engender so much passion, debate and excitement (Social Trends 1994).

Public sector leisure

Leisure activities provided by the public sector tend perhaps to be less flamboyant, invite more active participation and are often subsidised, so cost less. They include use of leisure centres and educational classes and sometimes focus on the public benefit. They also include provision of public space such as parks. Many now, however, tender out to the private sector for provision and maintenance.

Akin in nature at least to public sector provision are the services which are offered by national organisations such as The National Trust or the National Parks Commissions, which have a dual function of providing public facilities and undertaking conservation work. They too link strongly with work because they offer people the opportunity on a voluntary basis to be involved in their work, which can be dirty and arduous but very rewarding. Some activities such as mountain rescue are difficult to categorise as either work or leisure.

Passive leisure pursuits

Television is watched by 98% of men and women and is consistently the most popular form of leisure activity. Viewing varies and is most popular in the working class but, on average, about 26 hours of television is watched per person per week. Peak viewing times are when the popular 'soaps' are transmitted (General Household Survey 1983, Social Trends 1994). Kelly (1995) opines that 'TV-watching may be relaxing and recuperative due to its low investment requirements'. There is a debate about how passive television watching really is, as it also provides interest, engagement with the topic, education, emotional involvement, discussion and common interest for people.

Spectator sports are particularly interesting to men, especially football, rugby and cricket which draw large crowds to matches and instil loyalty and fervour. Other sports such as tennis, bowls, snooker and athletics draw considerable television audiences, as do special events such as the Olympic games. Reading is a pastime particularly but not exclusively enjoyed by women, although both sexes read newspapers. Gambling is indulged in by both sexes but in different ways.

Active leisure pursuits

The most popular active pursuit enjoyed by both sexes and all ages is walking. Other popular sports activities are swimming, snooker, keep fit, cycling, darts, golf and tenpin bowling. Running, soccer and badminton are popular amongst people below the age of 30 (General Household Survey 1990). Other active pastimes are gardening and do-it-yourself, enjoyed particularly by men, and craft work enjoyed by women. Minority interests focus on developing or practising expertise, such as participation in local orchestras and choirs, photographic or art clubs and more solitary activities such as bird-watching or collecting things.

In Britain, visiting the pub for social interaction is popular with both sexes and all age groups including people below the age of 18. Pubs vary in nature and may attract different customers such as certain age groups, men, families, gays and lesbians, working class and middle class, people working in specific occupations, single people and couples. They also offer activities, entertainment, music and food. They are an acceptable place for both meeting people and pursuing specific interests such as local political party meetings, musical interest groups, or meetings of charitable organisations.

The first half of this chapter has focused on a description and analysis of contemporary leisure patterns to explain the place, function and benefit of leisure time and to illustrate the range of pursuits which are available. The second half will concentrate on occupational therapy, leisure and acute mental illness or ill health.

OCCUPATIONAL THERAPY, LEISURE AND MENTAL ILL HEALTH

Occupational therapy is the therapeutic use of purposeful activity to improve a person's daily living function and enable that person to be as independent as is possible and appropriate, in the most suitable environment. The occupational therapist works with the patient, client or service user in an enabling capacity to assist him or her to achieve a chosen and maximum ability. The strength of occupational therapy is that it focuses for the most part on ordinary, banal, everyday living experiences. The power of the occupational therapist's skill is in the ability to use and develop a person's potential, strengths and skills to participate in banal, everyday living experiences. Activities of daily living include self-care, domestic activities and mobility. The pursuit of these activities is well documented in professional texts. Work is another everyday living pursuit which has engaged occupational therapists over time, although in a fluctuating pattern. Leisure, which as the preceding discussion illustrates is an accepted part of everyday living, tends to be less discussed in great detail by therapists, although they have always claimed it to be within their work remit. Why there is a relative paucity of work done on leisure is difficult to understand, particularly as we use so many activities that are commonly associated with leisure, such as craft work, art, horticulture and cooking, to promote a feeling of well-being.

Leisure and its concomitant satisfactory mental state could be made more available within regular occupational therapy programmes that are offered to people with problems associated with mental ill health or illness. The rationale lies in the core belief that people are occupational beings with an interest in being active and involved within their environment, but who may experience occupational dysfunction and consequent stress which may be relieved by participation in appropriate and acceptable occupation (Kielhofner 1992). This rationale fits the occupational therapist's involvement in leisure as well as activities of daily living and work. Well people living in the community indulge in leisure pursuits of various kinds; people with mental health problems are part of that community and for them to indulge in leisure pursuits is normal, a right and therapeutic. It is the occupational therapist's remit to assist functional living and, therefore, to address leisure is a professional responsibility which should not be neglected.

Some of the short-term mental health or illness problems which occupational therapy service users may manifest are depression, anxiety, schizophrenia in its acute stages, obsessive–compulsive disorders, eating disorders, phobias, post-traumatic stress syndrome, abnormal manifestations of illness and unacceptable levels of stress (Goldberg et al 1994). These may be due to biochemical imbalances, trauma such as acquired brain injury, or psychosocial difficulties such as those associated with underemployment, unemployment, redundancy, retirement, acting as a long-term carer, financial difficulties, poor social skills, social upheaval, bereavement, feelings of inadequacy or unsatisfactory personal relationships. Problems manifest themselves in behavioural and cognitive disorders, low self-esteem, extreme stress, poor functional skills, inadequate coping skills, poor cognitive skills, withdrawal, avoidance behaviour, aggression and dependency.

Some people with mental health problems will be employed in paid work, others will have family responsibilities. Others will have neither of these and will have poorly defined social roles and lack structure in their lives. Many people will have much time on their hands but will not experience a feeling of well-being because of it. Grint (1991) discusses the negative implications of unemployment which suitably describes the state of having time but no enjoyment of it. He claims that 'unemployment appears to rob the unemployed of the resources and will to undertake any kind of constructive activity' and destroys routine, social networks and status.

The Model of Human Occupation (Kielhofner 1992) is a useful tool to analyse some of the difficulties people may have in successfully partaking in leisure activities. According to Kielhofner, the human person is conceptualised as an open system subject to input, throughput, output and feedback. Problems regarding leisure may occur at any one of these points. The occupational therapist has the knowledge and skill to assess and locate difficulties. A key consideration may be the environment in which the person lives, where unsatisfactory relationships, lack of knowledge, facilities or money may prevent access to leisure. Intake of information into the system may be further impeded by poorly functioning sensory, perceptual or cognitive abilities which block adequate or positive stimulation. Throughput may be affected in any one of the three subsystems of volition, habituation and performance. The person may lack the motivation, interest, adaptability or energy to seek out, develop or participate in leisure pursuits, or have negative beliefs about his or her level of control or personal skills. These difficulties will impede the performance skills necessary for the accomplishment of constructive activity. Kielhofner's model offers the therapist a useful tool to use in the analysis of a person's leisure problems. Another form of assessment which may be used is the Assessment of Motor and Process Skills (AMPS).

A health promotion approach may shift the emphasis away

from a problem focus to one of improving health through involvement in leisure pursuits. For some clients this may be an enticing and acceptable approach within the remit of primary and secondary health promotion (Ewles & Simnett 1992) as it emphasises normal health and is familiar to the population at large through the media. It is associated with topical, well-advertised physical issues such as limiting smoking and drinking and eating well. It lacks the stigma which may be associated with more therapeutic approaches. For others, a simple problem-solving model may be appropriate to focus on self-identified problems such as loneliness or lack of exercise. A rehabilitation model will emphasise the re-acquisition of lost leisure skills and an educational model will target learning new skills. All of these different theoretical perspectives offer the therapist and service user a choice of approaches and methods of working to suit different needs. The therapist who can analyse and practise using alternate frames of reference, models or approaches has a much wider repertoire of knowledge and skills with which to access solutions.

OCCUPATIONAL THERAPY AND LEISURE PROGRAMMES

A series of possible programmes will be discussed which refer to the different issues already raised, such as variables that affect leisure, different types of leisure, mental health problems and theoretical approaches that influence practice, in order to bring together the many aspects of this topic. All these programmes may be offered within an acute psychiatric inpatient service, a day hospital, a community mental health programme or the client's local and home environment.

Hobby groups

A number of occupational therapy departments work within a simple easy-to-manage structure which focuses on the main difficulties associated with mental illness or ill health. They tend to adopt an uncomplicated but effective problem-solving approach which targets specific life skills, such as stress or anxiety management, home management and cooking, keep fit, confidence building, self-assertiveness skills or self-presentation. A regular programme may be organised and people allocated to groups depending on their interest or advice from staff. They require active participation and will centre on the activity rather than on any psychodynamic processes.

Hobby groups may be part of this repertoire. A number of activities may be chosen which could be adapted to suit different levels of skills. People assessed as having inadequate leisure pursuits may be invited to attend. The groups will usually relate to specific activities such as woodwork, painting, photography, pottery, dressmaking or cookery. They may be run by occupational therapists, support workers, technical instructors or craft experts. The standard of work varies depending on the skills of the staff and the interest, ability and motivation of participants. Involvement is often short term and little evaluation has been done on the carry-over of interest after discharge. They are effective, however, in engaging some people in active participation, particularly at a time of crisis when life is difficult. They can also provide symptom relief for varying lengths of time from preoccupation and wearying thoughts. A successful outcome produces a feeling of well-being which in itself is therapeutic but the number of people who develop new leisure activities as a result of these groups has never been fully recorded.

Special interest leisure groups

Akin to the above, but more structured and formally organised, are therapy sessions which focus on one activity, often led by someone who has a special skill or interest in that area. Their purpose is not necessarily to use the activity for a significant reason such as nonverbal expression or role play, as art therapy or drama therapy sessions may, but to participate actively in a normal, pleasurable pastime. They differ from adult education sessions in that the person running them has knowledge and understanding of both the activity and the special problems that members may have and, therefore, can facilitate involvement and group cohesion.

A simple and effective format is that used by Inglis (1993), who organised a 'reading for pleasure' group using her expertise as a librarian. She wished to offer mentally ill people 'a leisure activity based on reading' which might provide 'a welcome alternative to television'. People were invited to the group and introduced to a pre-selected or self-selected array of books which were read aloud, perused and discussed. No formal analysis of the outcome was made but people attended freely and some looked forward to and enjoyed the sessions. No doubt, much of the success was related to good organisation, careful choice of books and the commitment of the person running the sessions.

Many therapists have special talents and interests such as music and dance qualifications, a love of cooking or sewing, knowledge of films or the theatre, or interesting hobbies such as collecting old photographs or the creative use of papier mâché. It is difficult to be accepted on a professional occupational therapy undergraduate course without some skill other than academic ability. By using these personal abilities combined with therapeutic skills, there is enormous potential for widening the scope of many service users' interests and occupational repertoire. Because of the nature of short-term community care, sessions may have to be freestanding and finite, but with a link to the next one for those who may attend for longer periods.

Self-support groups

Self-support groups meet because the members have a common problem which the group collectively understands and can support from within. Social contact is one provision. Other groups meet primarily for social or leisure contact; an example is the Outsiders Club for people who have become socially isolated, which is organised nationwide by its members (Oliveck 1995). It is advantageous if occupational therapists have knowledge of and, preferably, personal links with support groups in order to inform people who may be interested and assist them to make contact.

Gender-based leisure groups

As discussed above, some leisure pursuits are of more interest to either men or women. Women tend to be more involved in home-based activities and craft work while men maintain an interest in sport, for example. Occupational therapists as part of their remit often assist gender-based self-support groups to establish themselves, particularly women's groups. This entails bringing a group of people together, establishing aims, finding an easily accessible community location, providing initial leadership, materials, information and support, and gradually withdrawing as the group matures. Contact is usually maintained and assistance made available when necessary or sought. The occupational therapist is also a referral source for new members.

Leisure should be a part of the group's agenda. A women's group may choose to undertake some home-based leisure activities such as making cakes for special occasions, or craft work. The group may offer mutual support for excursions into the wider community, to the cinema, an exhibition or the leisure centre. Chosen pursuits may focus on self-presentation through discussion of clothes, colours or make-up, or alternatively on the house by consideration of home decoration on a low budget. Family-based leisure may be supported by the group, particularly for those members who are single parents in that family excursions can be arranged to provide supportive social contact and assistance to both parents and children.

Men's groups for people who have short-term mental health problems are less common. There are men's groups in the wider community, however, who meet as a male company such as in Rotary Clubs or at working men's clubs, so the principal is established. Some groups, by the nature of the problem in focus, may be all male, however; for example those associated with AIDS and the mental health problems which can result. Leisure pursuits to facilitate a feeling of well-being and pleasurable state of mind are advantageous. The occupational therapist's role is more likely to be that of enabler than leader because the members are less likely to have had former experience of potentially disabling mental health problems and will have had intact social lives.

Common leisure pursuits

The most common leisure pursuits among the general population are home-centred, involving craft work, family leisure, do-it-yourself activities, watching television, listening to the radio, especially music, watching videos, playing tapes or compact discs or taking days out or going on holiday. These are normal, banal, frequently experienced pursuits. If a major function of the occupational therapist's role is to make the banal available, then there is clearly a wealth of activities at hand to form the base of comfortable leisure pursuits.

The most habitual common pastime is watching television. The most popular viewing time is early evening when the long-running soap operas are transmitted. It would be a truly imaginative development to use television viewing as a focus for some leisure sessions. The aim, of course, would be to introduce some degree of creative selection and points of interest to television watching and perhaps, if agreed by participants, to reduce the hours of non-selective viewing. As Kelly (1995) has indicated, television does stimulate conversation, provides entertainment and company, facilitate shared family time, and can be educational if this is a desired goal. Sessions on television watching could involve:

- analysis of current watching patterns and the reasons why they occur
- exposure to different types of programmes
- discussion of whether or not people wish to reduce watching time and how to do it.

Television watching can also be the focus of day trips to studios or locations associated with popular shows.

Taking a holiday is a normal pursuit and an occupational therapist would be advantaged if she or he had knowledge of different types of holidays or could stimulate discussion to enable clients, patients or service users to share holiday experiences. Some people may have difficulty in organisation of holidays, selecting within a budget or, more fundamentally, allowing themselves the opportunity to take a holiday. Holiday discussions could be linked with television travel and holiday programmes which offer information on a wide variety of locations and prices.

Low-budget leisure pursuits

Those people with short-term mental illness or mental health problems who do not work or are underemployed will have budgetary constraints which obviously must be taken into consideration. Leisure activities have a strong consumer element about them and many require excess income for participation. However, some cost less or nothing at all. The occupational therapist should have a broad local knowledge of available low-cost leisure opportunities.

Watching television and listening to the radio are obvious choices. Television watching has already been discussed. Most radio listening involves listening to music, but a common leisure pursuits group may explore a wider selection of channels and types of programmes, including those relating to other interests such as serialisations of plays and books and specialist broadcasts relating to gardening or family life. Public libraries and museums were established for people on low incomes, and other public facilities such as leisure centres have special concessionary rates for the unemployed and older user.

Another relatively low-cost activity is concern for and interest in animals. Dogs in particular have a very high capacity for unconditional positive regard but not all people will be able or willing to give the commitment required to keep one, in spite of the calming and companionship benefits of dog ownership. An interest in urban wildlife and, particularly, urban bird-watching and -feeding is absorbing, however. Horticulture is another relatively low-cost interest, and specialist interest leisure groups could assist in the organisation of knowledge, materials and equipment required to set up home-based small projects. As with cooking, there is a plethora of cheap literature on gardening in libraries, supermarkets and magazines, which could inform such groups. Feeding oneself is a necessary everyday function but the pursuit of variety within the diet could be advantageously encouraged.

Age-related leisure groups

This particular discussion will focus on the elderly, even though the principle of special groups for different ages is general. Many elderly service users with functional disorders may be experiencing unpleasant social sequelae such as isolation, loneliness, dejection, poor physical health and limited concentration. The habitual programme which occupational therapists and other care workers turn to is reminiscence therapy. This is beneficial but there is much scope for the introduction of more varied programmes, including those related to leisure pursuits. Dancing, swimming and walking can all be done using different energy and ability levels and have the added bonus of improving muscle strength and blood circulation, and reducing the rate of bone density loss. Libraries have an ever-improving selection of large-print books as well as records, tapes and compact discs which can be borrowed. Another source of pleasure for those with video machines, is the wide variety of tapes that is available of beautiful scenery and melodious songs which uplift the mood and are difficult not to sing along with. Occupational therapists are advantaged if they have knowledge of facilities available locally which are suitable for older clients, and the clientele are advantaged if the occupational therapist can be forward thinking as well as being knowledgeable about reminiscence.

Leisure management

A sound programme to develop would be a leisure management programme. There are well-established stress and anxiety management programmes available to provide a model. The programme should have the following:

- clearly defined aims and goals
- a set structure, time limit and schedule
- a defined client group
- a location
- a knowledgeable leader and/or enabler.

The group ethos should use or combine rehabilitation, habilitation, problem-solving and health-promotion approaches as appropriate to enable the re-establishment of old leisure pursuits, teach new ones and offer exploration of and practice in different kinds of leisure activities in order to improve the mental health of its members.

PROBLEMS RELATING TO LEISURE THERAPY PROGRAMMES

These problems are not necessarily exclusive to leisure provision. General problems relate to:

- lack of client interest, which may be a symptom of mental stress and therefore requires analysis
- lack of interest from other staff who have their own work to do and therefore inadvertently may block development
- lack of space and resources
- lack of initiative, interest or knowledge by the occupational therapist.

Addressing these problems

The first problem which should be addressed is the occupational therapist's limitations and level of commitment. If a commitment is made, the therapist needs to develop a knowledge and resource base on local leisure opportunities and widen his or her knowledge of the subject of leisure in general so that provision can be offered from a solid, psychosocial information base. Problems relating to other staff commitment or interest should be analysed and discussed and difficulties addressed because they prevent quality provision of service. All programmes, be they simple hobby groups or a formal leisure management programme, should be discussed and planned with clear aims and objectives. Therapists may find it useful to learn some basic marketing techniques to present these to other staff and service users. Knowledge, careful organisation and appropriate marketing should increase the success of any initiative.

CONCLUSION

Occupational therapists have skills in all aspects of the occupational therapy process. They have available an increasing source of theoretical and practical knowledge and developments to draw upon. They have personal skills and interests and the ability to seek out and acquire new ones. They know how to resource, organise and use information including the background information of the subject in question. They also understand the importance of environment and enablement. Leisure is a neglected area in occupational therapy but therapists have all the skills to make it a vibrant and interesting one. Leisure induces a feeling of well-being, relaxation or stimulation. These are psychosocial experiences which are advantageous to people with short-term mental illness or mental health problems. Occupational therapists therefore have a professional responsibility and aptitude to develop this area of their work.

REFERENCES

Bond J, Bond S 1994 Sociology and health care, 2nd edn, Churchill Livingstone, Edinburgh
Bond J, Coleman P, Peace S (eds) 1993 Ageing in society, 2nd edn. Sage Publications, London
Clarke J, Critcher C 1995 Coming home to roost. In: Critcher C, Bramham P, Tomlinson A (eds) Sociology of leisure—a reader. E & F N Spon, London
Ewles L, Simnett I 1992 Promoting health. Scutari Press, London
General Household Survey 1983 HMSO, London
General Household Survey 1990 HMSO, London
Giddens A 1993 Sociology, 2nd edn. Polity Press, Cambridge

Green E, Hebron S, Woodward D 1995 Women's leisure today. In: Critcher C, Bramham P, Tomlinson A (eds) Sociology of leisure—a reader. E & F N Spon, London
Grint K 1991 The sociology of work. Polity Press, Cambridge
Goldberg D, Benjamin S, Creed F 1994 Psychiatry in medical practice, 2nd edn. Routledge, London
Hardy T 1874 Far from the madding crowd. Penguin Books, England
Inglis J 1993 Reading for pleasure: an experiment using fiction with psychiatric patients. British Journal of Occupational Therapy 56(7): 258–261
Kelly J R 1995 Leisure and the family. In: Critcher C, Bramham P, Tomlinson A (eds) Sociology of leisure—a reader. E & F N Spon, London
Kielhofner G 1992 Conceptual foundations of occupational therapy. F A Davis, Philadelphia
Oliveck M 1995 Inside story. Therapy Weekly 21(34): 4
Parker S 1976 The sociology of leisure. George Allen and Unwin, London
Roberts K 1995 Great Britain: socioeconomic polarisation and the implications for leisure. In: Critcher C, Bramham P, Tomlinson A (eds) Sociology of leisure—a reader. E & F N Spon, London
Social Trends 24 1994 HMSO, London
Veblen T 1899 The theory of the leisure class

FURTHER READING

Finlay L 1988 Occupational therapy practice in psychiatry. Chapman & Hall, London
Leisure Studies (Journal of). E & F N Spon, London
Young M E, Quinn E 1992 Theories and Principles of Occupational Therapy. Churchill Livingstone, Edinburgh

Family therapy

Becky Durant

INTRODUCTION

Occupational therapists work within a number of specialist multi-disciplinary teams, each involving a broadening or redefinition of professional role and each relating to a different set of theoretical problems. Working with families provides a useful example of one such area of practice. The following account illustrates the tensions and choices which may confront a therapist and outlines emerging theoretical themes which influence therapy.

Family therapy was born in the 1950s of mixed parentage. After 30 years and still pubescent it found a place in many child and family centres where, for a number of occupational therapists, it has superseded play therapy as a major technique.

Throughout its journey, family therapy has refined and transformed itself into one of the most commonly chosen techniques in family centres. This chapter describes how this change has taken place and the implications for occupational therapists.

Traditionally, occupational therapists were responsible for individual work with children and adolescents, primarily using play therapy techniques. Doctors interviewed parents, psychologists psychometrically tested children and social workers were responsible for family work. So, many people were involved, each person doing his or her bit, but rarely meeting together with the family or with each other.

The child was viewed as the problem and probably given a label to reinforce both this view and the need for individual work. In fact there were many diagnostic criteria from which to choose, from adjustment reaction to conduct disorder and from elimination problems to eating difficulties. The child and family centres' primary task was to treat the child in order to get rid of the problem.

This somewhat linear and reductionist approach lasted until the late 1970s, when there was a shift in focus from a cause-and-effect model, to a circular, systemic paradigm. The individual child was no longer the focus of attention; instead, the whole family was seen as a 'system' and each individual family member as an important part of that system. Indeed the word 'system' became very fashionable until the late 1980s when it grew and became 'systemic'.

The language of therapy changed to embrace a burgeoning of new concepts, many of these arising from the work of Bertalanffy (1950), the founder of general systems theory.

The western world has dozens of family therapy journals and the flood of literature shows little sign of abating. Many institutions offer courses in family therapy and some are forming links with universities to strengthen the research base of the technique. The future may require British family therapists to register as 'psychotherapists' before they can practice, as this is the current situation in most European countries.

THE EMERGENCE OF FAMILY THERAPY

Many professionals, including occupational therapists, have gradually adopted the title of family therapists. Indeed, it seemed more appropriate for the families to receive appointment letters from family therapists than occupational therapists. Therefore multidisciplinary units could be redefined as 'not so multi-disciplinary' as most workers took on this new identity.

A blurring of roles emerged and preciousness over disciplines began to disappear. Perhaps the advent of family therapy helped to improve relationships between different professions as some of the traditional jealousy began to evaporate.

The rapid growth in the field of family therapy can be compared to the development of psychoanalysis at the turn of the century. If, in psychoanalysis, it was difficult for the clinician to define his or her concepts clearly, the task for the family therapist was even more daunting. But this became a shared task for all the professions irrespective of background or training.

Learning the language

It is difficult to find a common language for family therapy as it arose from the work of a number of people. It was and is the brainchild of several creative therapists and investigators, many of whom were and are in close contact with each other. Several ideas and concepts were developed, often meaning the same thing but called something else. To add to the richness, the proponents of family therapy came from a number of different theoretical and practical backgrounds. They arose from backgrounds in psychoanalysis, social work, sociology, psychiatry and anthropology. I do not think that there was a representative from the field of occupational therapy. Each discipline brought its different wealth of experience and, most importantly, its different ways of speaking about that experience. These diverse backgrounds included information theory, general systems theory, communication theory, cybernetics theory (from the world of Dr Who) as well as linguistics, biology, psychopathology and others.

Therapists started to view families in a different way; as an interactional system that operated according to rules and principles that apply to all systems.

They were united in their newly acquired professional beliefs about circular causality or nonsummativity. These words, with particular meaning, were added to each therapist's vocabulary and almost overnight a new language was born.

Circular causality is a subtle move from seeing causes as linear to appreciating them as circular. Families were redefined as a group of individuals interrelated so that a change in any one member affects other individuals and the family as a whole. Cause and effect are interchangeable. They are events within a sequence and to select one or more of these events may completely miss the point. In fact, what is 'cause' one minute is 'effect' the next.

This new way of thinking challenges traditional thoughts and, to an extent, the medical model. Traditionally, therapists subscribe to the idea that certain causes lead, in linear fashion, to certain effects. This dilemma about definition is paralleled by a difference between western and eastern thought. In western thinking, a positivistic approach is adopted which describes something as 'is' or 'is not'. Something is either hot or cold, fat or thin. It cannot be both at once. But in eastern thinking it can be. Its definition may be dependent on its relation to other processes or entities.

This non-linear paradigm may have posed a problem for many present-day research methods and statistical tools. Indeed, non-linear research proposals are often rejected by non-family therapy reviewers.

Nonsummativity was also added to the therapist's vocabulary. Its meaning is less unfamiliar than its pronunciation—the whole is greater than the sum of its parts. Or, in the case of therapy, the family is greater than the sum of its parts. Its parts are its individual members. The idiosyncratic behaviours of individual members cannot be added up to describe the family. Instead, the family organisation and interactional patterns involve an interlocking of the actions and behaviour of the individuals within it. The therapist and family need to look at the patterns that emerge and the connections between the actions and behaviours of the family members.

Communication (which later becomes 'cybernetics') replaced the word 'behaviour'. All communication transmits interpersonal messages and has two functions. The first is to convey information and the second to convey how the information is to be taken, and thus it defines the relationship. Family systems stabilise the process of defining relationships through family rules. Family rules became another extension of the therapist's vocabulary. These family rules determine the family lifestyle.

There are other terms, such as 'homeostasis', that ascended within the literature and then lost favour almost as quickly as they were introduced. Others, however, including those mentioned above, have been grouped and are used to describe specific models of family therapy. The interested reader can refer to any book on family therapy for further definitions and knowledge. Some of these terms have disappeared and reappeared with slightly different meanings during the evolution of family therapy.

Structure and strategy

An important contribution was made in the work of Salvador Minuchin (1974) whose name became synonymous with structural family therapy. Many occupational therapists were greatly influenced by his ideas. This type of therapy is concerned with family organisation and the part it plays in the functioning of the family unit and the subsequent health of its individual family members. It is based, therefore, on the normative concept of a healthy functioning family with healthy members. Concepts such as boundaries and hierarchies are often used with this technique. Particular emphasis is placed upon the boundaries between family subsystems and the establishment of a clear hierarchy, with parents at the top making all the final decisions. A structurally oriented therapist assesses the dysfunctional structures in the family such as blurred boundaries, confused family hierarchies and maybe the existence of rigid coalitions. The therapist uses a variety of techniques to restructure the boundaries, and it is hoped that new patterns will develop which are more effective in problem solving.

Occupational therapists are generally creative by nature and can find that they have an ability to teach families more effective problem-solving skills. This theoretical base also instilled in therapists some confidence, instead of the usual apprehension and fear that accompanies new expectations and foreign ground.

Occupational therapists working within this framework derived both satisfaction and recognition. They possessed the relevant skills to observe and identify a malfunctioning family and could be instrumental in making the family members more aware of their maladaptive pattern.

Other therapists progressed to an interest in strategic family therapy. Again there is some overlap with the structuralists, sharing vocabulary such as 'hierarchies' and 'boundaries'. It too is a very directive form of therapy. Here, similarly to structural family therapy, family problems are seen as the expression of dysfunctional organisational patterns such as blurred generational boundaries or confusions in the family hierarchy. Together with the family, goals of therapy are negotiated and then a strategy is outlined to achieve the goals.

Strategic therapy differs from structural therapy in that more emphasis is placed on the functional aspect of symptoms. In other words, therapists consider the symptoms and ask themselves questions such as: 'What function does this symptom serve for this family or this individual?' or 'How can this symptom be replaced by something else that serves the same purpose?'

Many strategic therapists work in a team using a one-way screen. The therapist sits in a room with the family and the rest of the team, with a nominated supervisor, sits the other side. Permission from the family is always sought and the family usually meet the team. The reason for the screen stems from the belief that during therapy a new, more or less coherent, system is created between the therapist and the family. The therapist in the room with the family has difficulty in maintaining an objective view of the family or new system of which he or she is a part.

The therapist attempts to change the family's patterns of communication and uses methods such as positive connotation of symptoms or paradoxical interventions.

Positive connotation refers to a therapist's positive evaluation of actions or behaviour that would usually be regarded as pathological. In this way confrontation is avoided between therapist and family and the family is encouraged to change its value system and view of the world. When the meaning of an action is altered, family members must necessarily react in a different manner towards this behaviour.

Paradoxical interventions involve exposing the family to contradictory instructions. For example, a therapist might suggest that the family should keep doing whatever it is they want to change. The therapist takes control of the therapeutic system. If the symptom continues, this can be viewed as compliance with the therapist. If the symptom disappears, then therapy can be viewed as successful. Paradoxical interventions aim at invalidating the family's own pathogenic paradoxes, which they have created from their own family beliefs. These techniques have been described by various authors especially Erickson & Rossi (1975).

The main difference between 'strategic' and 'structural' orientations can be seen by comparing each style's foci. The former has a communicational focus on problems and the latter pays attention to the sociological structures of family systems.

The sociological structure of the family system is conceived by structuralists in terms of subsystem units, such as wife–husband, father–child, and siblings. When a family is too enmeshed or lacking in subsystem differentiation, things may go wrong. The purpose of structural family therapy is to help differentiate and connect subsystems.

Structural and strategic therapists can be seen as starting in opposite directions. The structuralists begin with a complete theoretical model of family structure. To a strategic therapist, on the other hand, the family's presenting problem leads to a view of the sequential pattern organising it and then to the semantic and political frames of social hierarchy and coalition patterns, respectively. Some strategic therapists use particular family problems as a lever for changing structures. As the structural therapist is primarily concerned with changing structure, the sequence embodying the presenting problem need not be addressed.

Structural therapists ask questions that sometimes construct a view that one person's problematic behaviour is related to other family members. This type of construction, familiar to so many family therapists, is actually the semantic frame of reference called 'family therapy'.

The more one tries to differentiate structure and strategy the more they appear to have in common. Perhaps this contributes to reasons for a move from strategic therapy to systemic therapy on the part of a number of occupational therapists.

Systemic therapy

Systemic therapy has developed rapidly over the past few years and has been influenced by sociology, anthropology and social psychology. Biology and physics, important early on, now fade into the background. The term systemic therapy is often used with reference to the Milan model of family therapy.

The Milan model of systemic therapy was developed by Mara Selvini Palazzoli and her co-workers. In 1967, the first centre for family therapy was created in Italy by Palozzoli and Luigi Boscolo. A group of 10 psychiatrists with a psychoanalytical bias towards their work met frequently to discuss cases. 4 years later, in 1971, a few of the original team left the psychoanalytical model and became interested in the interactional model. These four, Selvini-Palazzoli, Boscolo, Gianfranco Cecchin and Guilina Prata became known as the 'Milan Team'.

From 1975, the team studied the theories proposed by Bateson (1972) and used them extensively in their work. Their work was also greatly influenced by the strategic school of family therapy and communication theory of Watzlawick and his colleagues (Watzlawick et al 1967).

Within these models, the family is viewed as a self-organising, cybernetic system in which all the elements are linked to one another and, as with strategic theory, the presenting problem of the family fulfils a specific function for the family system. Systemic theory looks at the wider context of the family including its social context. The referring agent or the child's school and the therapeutic team itself are considered as potentially important elements of the system and are considered in therapy as well as the family.

Usually, attention is paid to the importance of hypothesising. Why has the family sought help now? What are the family's expectations? What are the goals the family hope to accomplish in the therapy? These initial hypotheses are examined or confirmed through a very special method of questioning called 'circular questioning' first introduced by Peggy Penn (1982).

Circular questioning is used to find out directly what a person thinks about someone or something else. It aims to gather information and at the same time introduce something new into the system. This gathering of information aids in the formulation and validation of hypotheses regarding the family's structure. As communication is largely about the behaviour of others, the dangers of self-referencing in response to questions are avoided. If, for example, in another therapy, a child is asked to comment about his or her relationship to a parent, the answer given in the presence of the parents becomes itself an element of that relationship. It may even consolidate or intensify an existing loyalty conflict. In circular questioning, it is possible indirectly to discuss family secrets or taboo subjects by using 'what if' questions. For example, one can respect the secret but ask about the possible consequences of disclosure and how people think other family members might react.

Many occupational therapists have noticed that this type of questioning can be very helpful in engaging children in therapy sessions. For many years, occupational therapists and other professionals have been operating with the belief that children find it very hard to verbalise, and respond better on a nonverbal level. This has led to the introduction of toys and pens and paper in the interviewing room, and hence the use of non-directive play therapy. The author believes that children will respond according to the expectations imposed upon them. If they walk into a room full of toys, they will naturally assume that the toys are for them and will start playing. A basket full of Lego is hardly likely to be there for their parents. But could they verbalise if given the correct opportunity?

Many educationalists have researched children and their ability to articulate (Wells 1986, Wray 1990). They have found that children are able to communicate at quite a young age, providing the questions and language chosen are suitable. It would appear that, although psychologists and other professions have much to contribute about general child development, they can also learn from educationalists who have specialised in children's language.

For instance, direct questions usually produce little response. Both educational literature and experience confirm this and have demonstrated that children are very good at describing what they have seen and in particular are good at talking about someone else. Children, when asked to comment about mummy's reaction when daddy does or says something, are usually very able to reply because they are good observers.

Generally speaking, there is a wealth of therapeutic literature on how to engage children on a nonverbal level, but very little about how to do this on a verbal level. However, there is plenty written about types of questioning, particularly in relation to systemic therapy. Few people, however, have actually made the connection between certain types of questioning and the effect this has on the child in therapy. Without realising it, systemic therapy has played a major part in enabling children to participate in sessions by giving them room to have a voice. The days of silencing them with toys are over!

REFLECTION ON PRACTICE

The introduction of systemic therapy generated a period of reflection and critical thinking. Many occupational therapists working as family therapists became aware of personal and professional beliefs and other factors that had influenced them in reaching their present position. The notion of neutrality, or suspending one's own feelings, in therapy became important. Many therapists believed it essential to become more in tune with their own feelings so that they could identify times when they were being influenced by factors outside the therapy room. Was their hypothesis really based on something the family had said or was it a result of an article they had recently read? How much was present-day fashionable thinking influencing their judgement?

Occupational therapists, together with other professionals, started debating the process of change. Whilst in the position of a structural or strategic therapist, the shared belief was that effective problem-solving skills could be taught. Even if this concept of instructive interaction were possible, how does the therapist come to understand the problem? Would one therapist's interpretation of the problem coincide with everyone else's? In fact, does the problem or system exist as an entity that can readily be observed?

The concept of the therapist as expert became a dubious notion. Does the therapist really know better than the client? Can the therapist 'make' the client change? If so, does the therapist 'know' how the client needs to change? Is the therapist gifted with some superior knowledge that puts him or her in a superior advantaged position above that of the client? Some therapists wondered if they had showed their clients more respect as 'play therapists' when they had given total responsibility for the direction of therapy sessions, and therefore for change, to the child.

In order to learn something new or to change one's way of thinking, something external needs to disturb or stimulate a person's inner world, which then enables the person to reflect on his or her own actions or thoughts. Changing and learning are closely connected. No-one can give someone else knowledge or 'change'; there has to be reflection and thought. Similarities began to emerge between therapist and families in therapy. During this quest to become better therapists, the therapists went through the same experience as the families they were treating. Both experienced a disturbance of expectations; therapists questioned their professional beliefs and the families questioned their family beliefs.

Therapists began to question meaning and understanding. Is it possible to understand the other person or only to understand what the other person is saying? Actual events and real people cannot be understood, only their language. Therapists had previously been creative exponents of systems views that focused on the impact of structural or strategic patterns of interactions in family groups. They now turned to a search for a language of meanings to express the impact of their therapeutic encounters.

It may be significant that this concern with semantic properties of systems is taking place in other contexts as well as family therapy. Oakley (1990) has used the pages of a cognitive journal to present an argument for the properties of narrative investigations when dealing with accounts of human intentionality. Alan Parry (1991) has used the term 'narrative paradigm therapy' to propose a different way of working with individuals.

The issue of control emerged during this reflection on narratives. Does the use of circular questioning put the therapist in the position of control? If questions rather than observations become the primary mode of collecting data is everything under the therapist's control?

Therapists who created hypotheses and then asked questions to test them out might have been guilty of imposing their own ideas indirectly. Perhaps they continued asking questions until they got the answer they wanted. It is possible that the therapists were imposing a structure and creating a hierarchy through words and through language?

Construction and meaning

Adopting a slightly different perspective, many therapists turned to social construction theory and were influenced by Hoffman (1990) who posited this view:

... evolving set of meanings that emerge unendingly from the interactions between people. These meanings are not skull-bound and may not exist inside what we think of as an individual 'mind'. They are part of a general flow of constantly changing narratives. Thus, the theory by-passes the fixity of the model of biologically based cognition, claiming instead that the development of concepts is a fluid process, socially derived.

Hoffman proposes a view of meanings as embodied in language. Anderson & Goolishan (1998, p. 372) offer a version of this linguistic formulation geared specifically to the theory and practice of family therapy:

Human systems are language-generating and, simultaneously, meaning-generating systems ... The therapeutic system is a linguistic system ... Therapy is a linguistic event that takes place in what we call a therapeutic conversation ... Change is the evolution of new meaning through dialogue.

Meaning is created in the act of speech and does not exist outside the linguistic system.

Within this framework, there are no 'real' external entities, only communicating and languaging human individuals ... Conversation—language and communication—is simply part of the hermeneutic struggle to reach understanding with those with whom we are in contact—language does not mirror nature; language creates the nature we know.

Family therapy is a way of finding new meanings; meaning and understanding do not exist before the utterances of language. Therapy becomes a method of developing, through dialogue, new themes and narratives. In collaboration with the family, the therapist helps to create new descriptions and stories. With Hoffman's account no particular meanings are enforced, no grand narratives of cure, but partial fragments of possible narrative lines.

The therapeutic interview is a performance text, as the post-modernist jargon has it. This text will take its shape according to the emergent qualities of the conversation that have inspired it, and will hopefully create an emancipatory dialogue rather than reinforce the oppressive or monolithic one that so often comes in the door...

In this type of encounter the therapist listens to a story and then collaborates with the family present to invent other stories or other meanings for the stories.

CURRENT DEVELOPMENTS

For some therapists these developments produced a temporary feeling of fragmentation, of the inability to stay with meanings. Family therapy theories change very quickly; as soon as one model is proposed, another emerges, but most theories are fairly easy to grasp and are often a refinement of a previous one. Hoffman's theory produces a feeling of temporary disintegration. The idea of being held together, in connection with others and with one's own history and future, almost disappears. If no-one is in control of him- or herself and nothing means anything other than its surface suggests, then we all become 'rootless' and meaning disappears.

As there is no access to any one 'truth' that can make sense of experience for all people at all times, then all the minor truths which we believe in also disappear. What about Einstein and Newton; do they become as unreliable as Father Christmas?

Another, slightly modified, theory emerged. Whether this was to make the therapist feel better or was the result of empirical research is an interesting debate.

Therapists reconsidered the notion of change and decided that therapeutic change is linked with taking in something new in such a way that the inner world of the subject is reconstituted. First there is the sense of disintegration, of falling apart or loss and maybe of something potentially out of control. This degraded state becomes intolerable and so change must take place. Then the system is extended to incorporate the therapist and a new system is created. Frosh (1991) writes: 'This provides the contest that makes it possible for the degraded inner state to be explored in an arena in which it can eventually become visible.'

The emerging family systems theories offer a way of opening family therapy to a more flexible engagement with people's perception of themselves and others. This is in conjunction with a concern for the linguistic constructions that make these perceptions communicable and vulnerable to change.

Constant movement

In present practice there are many ways of conducting family therapy sessions. Some therapists have become 'eclectic' and adopt a different model according to the family's problem. Others use the word 'eclectic' to describe the amalgamation of techniques from more than one school of thought. Some will argue that all family therapy is eclectic as it has developed from several theories simultaneously from many different countries and it is impossible to identify the pure therapeutic base.

Perhaps one thing is certain. When the occupational therapists moved from working with the individual to working with the family system, they were simply moving one 'objectively treatable' structure from the individual system to the family system!

Now they can say that, if a treatable structure exists, it exists through language. And also they can say that this is their belief which they may share with many others of similar beliefs.

It might be helpful to interpret the development of family therapy in Kuhn's terms, by seeing it as a succession of 'revolutions' in which dominant paradigms are overthrown and replaced (Kuhn 1970). A 'paradigm' embodies the particular conceptual framework through which the community of therapists operate; through which their particular interpretation of 'reality' or beliefs is generated. It also incorporates models of enquiry or sets of techniques which ensure that any theoretical knowledge that is produced will be consistent with that view of reality that the paradigm supports.

The move from individual to family therapy and the various moves within family therapy itself emerged because of a discontent with an existing paradigm. Once faith is lost, debates are initiated and alternative paradigms emerge. Existing paradigms were overthrown or abandoned and new ones developed. These new paradigms attracted allegiance and supportive systems for the therapists, and better ways of treating families developed.

This paradigm shift in Kuhn's words was not based on systematic, logical or rational assessment of rival alternatives. It was not based on any appeal to reason. It was a scientific revolution brought about by the conversion of the research community or, in this case, the family therapists.

Kuhn talks about 'revolutions' but equally important is the concept of evolution. The many ideas and paradigms that have been described are evolving paradigms that seem attractive at the time. Family therapy will continue to change and occupational therapists working in child and family centres will also change their ideas and beliefs.

The world of family therapy is not stagnant. It was born in the early 1950s; 40 years later it is in its adolescence and perhaps in 40 years time it will still be youthful.

REFERENCES

Anderson H, Goolishan H 1988 Human systems as linguistic systems. Preliminary and evolving ideas about the implications for clinical theory. Family Process 27: 371–394

Bateson G 1972 Steps to an ecology of mind. Ballantine Books, New York

Bertalanffy L von 1950 The theory of open systems in physics and biology. Science 3: 23–29

Erickson M H, Rossi E 1975 Varieties of a double bind. American Journal of Hypnosis 17: 143–157

Frosh S 1991 The semantics of therapeutic change. Journal of Family Therapy 13(2): 183

Hoffman L 1990 Constructing realities. An art of lenses. Family Process 29: 1–12

Kuhn T S 1970 The structure of scientific revolution. University of Chicago Press, Chicago

Minuchin S 1974 Families and family therapy. Tavistock, London

Oakley K 1990 Freud's cognitive psychology of intention: the case of Dora. Mind and Language 5: 69–86

Parry A 1991 A universe of stories. Family Process 30 (March): 37–53

Penn P 1982 Circular questioning. Family Process 21: 267–280

Selvini-Palazzoli 1972 Paradox and counter paradox. A new model in the therapy of the family in schizophrenic transaction. Ballantine Books, New York

Selvini-Palazzoli 1980 Hypothesising—circularity—neutrality. Three guidelines for the conductor of the session. Family Process 19: 3–12

Soper P H, L'Abate L 1977 Paradox as a therapeutic technique: a review. International Journal of Family Counselling 5: 10–21

Watzlawick P, Beavin J H, Jackson D D 1967 Pragmatics of human communication. A study of interactional patterns, pathologies and paradoxes. W W Norton, New York

Wells G 1986 Meaning makers. Hodder & Stoughton Educational, London

Wray D (ed) 1990 Emerging partnerships: current research in language and literacy. Bera Dialogues. Multilingual Matters, Clevedon

12

Strategic skills

Michael Willson

INTRODUCTION

The work of an occupational therapist is not restricted to time spent with the defined patient: a large part of the day is spent working with colleagues. This time includes departmental meetings, meetings with other members of the treatment team, case conferences and other events. The role of the individual includes relating to others who are more senior and also to those for whom one is responsible. This latter group may include helpers who may have many years of experience but little formal training and also students from different disciplines.

Whilst the phenomenology in inter- and intraprofessional relationships is usually only latent, it seems useful, nevertheless, to identify a few frameworks and strategic skills to ensure perfect satisfaction from such interactions. The material in this chapter goes only part of the way to attaining this goal, lack of space restricting academic discussion of the issues involved. Much of what follows will be familiar and may ring certain bells in the reader who recognises past experiences and rules of thumb. I hope that the experience of seeing it set out on paper by someone else will be of interest and use. This is, therefore, a practical guide to the conduct of meetings, negotiations, decision making and the exertion of influence.

MEETINGS

A surprising proportion of working time is spent in meetings. Meetings come in all shapes and sizes and for a wide variety of purposes. A characteristic of most meetings is that the participants resent being there and do not feel that the meeting meets their goals and needs. However, meetings are crucial in the coordination and planning of work and 'meeting skills' are a legitimate professional acquisition for the occupational therapist.

It is useful to ask what is the actual purpose of each meeting—is it to collect information, to disseminate information, to plan projects, to provide support, to make decisions or to allow people to sound off? Is the meeting structured in such a way that these goals can be achieved? Are the necessary people present? Are there people present whose time is being wasted? It is really the chairman's duty to organise and structure the meeting, to ensure that the appropriate people are present for the relevant periods, and also to attend to the process of the meeting and keep it healthy and alive. It is, however, important that each and every member is clear about his role and duties, and how to use the meeting, if he is to achieve whatever it is that justifies him spending time at the meeting.

Meetings as group events

Meetings are special group events in which there is often too little time to properly attend to the inevitable group process. The following frameworks are succinct enough to be used in the busiest of meetings.

A psychologist, William Schutz, suggests that groups can be said to develop through three main processes:

1. *Inclusion.* A cluster of people congregate together and, whilst on the surface they will be discussing all sorts of things, the underlying theme is 'Do I belong? Do I want to belong? Do I want to belong if Sue Smith is involved?'. After a while and a certain amount of coming and going, an understanding about membership develops and the group can be said to have worked through its inclusion to establish a tentative—and fragile—boundary around it.

2. *Control.* The next theme is one of negotiating the norms and allegiances (amongst birds only is this the 'pecking order').

Members seek to check out the rules of the group such as how deeply will certain matters be discussed. This is done by almost invisible giving and denying of approval to comments that are too deep or too superficial for the comfort of the others. Meanwhile, members are checking out where they stand with other members and trying to find out how far they can depend on different people and whom they are prepared to support. After a while the group may reach an implicit agreement over the rules and allegiances and can be said to have established a first and tentative degree of trust through working through the control theme. The group then moves on to the third stage in which people know where they stand in this group and can get on with the work in hand, rather than feeling obliged to be sorting out their own personal relationships. This third stage is known as:

3. *Affect*. Feeling included and trustful, people can express and use their feelings, in a constructive and almost selfless way. The reader will be familiar with the working through of inclusion at many an event; control themes are most blatantly illustrated by the way in which a group of children start acting up and causing trouble just at the point when you thought that they were starting to get together. 'Control' can also be detected in the game playing, teasing or 'horseplay' or general testing out that goes on in groups of adults. When the membership of a group—or meeting—changes, the inclusion will be re-negotiated and the modified patterns of allegiance and possible shifts in norms have to be checked through before the group can return to working at the 'affect' stage. The cycle is also repeated if a group stays together for a while and the members want to make the intensity of involvement greater. For instance, a group of lads may have formed a functioning group in which to spend their evenings, but one day one of them says that he is short of money so how about they all go and rob the Post Office. At this point some of the lads may want to step out of the group (and maybe other lads join in) as the inclusion is re-negotiated. Then the group will turn to the control issues and negotiate the new norms: Will they use violence? Will they not betray their friends if caught? They will also check out their allegiances to make sure that they can trust each other in the group (about 30% of solved crime is solved because someone 'grasses').

In a meeting it is important that everyone experiences a welcome and a gesture of inclusion—especially when it is likely that they do not really wish to be there at all. It is also necessary to permit a few minutes for the control themes to be worked through in a covert fashion so that people feel that they have made their gesture and established their presence. This may take only 5 minutes before the business can get started but, if it is ignored, these personal issues will be being worked through at the expense of, and under the cover of, the item being discussed; the outcome of the case conference becomes less to do with the patient's condition and more to do with the score in the game of 'get the nurse/consultant/OT etc.'.

Schutz's framework is a quick way of working out where a group has reached. A second framework serves as a guide to what one can then do about it.

Task and maintenance

It is possible to consider behaviour in groups under the heading of either task behaviour or maintenance behaviour. Task behaviour is conduct which furthers the (defined) work of the group. Maintenance behaviour, on the other hand, is conduct that helps the group function productively. The model is derived from industrial production where, for instance, we are concerned with a drilling machine: task behaviour is drilling holes whilst maintenance behaviour is stripping it down, oiling it and so on. The optimum balance is where the maintenance behaviour is sufficient but not in excess of what is necessary to permit the task to be achieved. Too much task focus and, although a lot of holes will be drilled in the short term, the machine burns out: too much maintenance behaviour and few holes are drilled even though a year later the machine is still immaculate.

Groups in which there is insufficient maintenance behaviour may achieve a great deal in the short term but they, too, burn out in the medium term. Groups in which there is insufficient task behaviour become cosy but boring and ineffective. Group members need to be attentive to the balance of task and maintenance behaviour, for otherwise the members will soon cease to get much satisfaction out of their membership.

Individuals have certain needs and requirements which are partially satisfied within a group. If the group is, in fact, a meeting, then these needs are both to achieve the goals of the meeting and also to fulfil simple personal needs such as occur in any social situation. If these needs are not being met, then the individual is very likely to give up on the group meeting. We can schematise this pattern in Table 12.1. In order that the group or meeting

Table 12.1 The needs and functions of a working group

Task needs of the group i.e. for a clear goal for agreement about goal for plan of action and so on	Must be met through task behaviour	Initiating Informing Clarifying Summarising Consensus	IF these are performed adequately
			AND
Maintenance needs of the group i.e. for mutual support for clarity for mutual understanding and so on	Must be met through maintenance behaviour	Harmonising Gate keeping Encouraging Compromising Giving feedback	these are performed adequately → THEN you have a good group!
			AND
Individual needs of the members i.e. to belong to be respected for status for power for dependency and so on	Must be met through group task and maintenance behaviour The residue manifests as personal or self-oriented behaviour	Aggressive behaviour Blocking Dominating Avoiding Abandoning	individual needs are met in the maintenance behaviour of the group

Table 12.2

Group task behaviour	Conduct that furthers the work of the group
1. Initiating	Proposes aims, ideas, actions or procedures
2. Informing	Asks for or offers facts, ideas, feelings or options
3. Clarifying	Illuminates or builds upon ideas or suggestions
4. Summarising	Pulls data together, so group may consider where it is
5. Consensus	Explores whether group may be nearing a decision; prevents premature decision making

Group maintenance behaviour	Conduct that helps the group function productively
1. Harmonising	Reconciles disagreements, relieves tension, helps people explore differences
2. Gate keeping	Brings others in, suggests facilitating procedures, keeps communication channels open
3. Encouraging	Is warm and responsive; indicates with words or facial expression that the contributions of others are accepted
4. Compromising	Modifies own positions so that group may move ahead; admits error
5. Giving feedback	Tells others, in helpful ways, how their behaviour is received

Personal or self-oriented behaviour	Conduct that interferes with the work of the group
1. Aggressive behaviour	Attacks, deflates, uses sarcasm
2. Blocking	Resists beyond reason, uses 'hidden agenda' items which prevent group movement
3. Dominating	Interrupts, asserts authority, over-participates to point of interfering with others' participation
4. Avoiding	Prevents group from facing controversy; stays off subject to avoid commitment
5. Abandoning	Makes an obvious display of lack of involvement

should be able to achieve its goals and to work well, the task and maintenance needs of the group must be met and, through the satisfaction of doing this, the individual needs of the members must be met. Table 12.2 illustrates how each and every person in a group can lead that group towards the attainment of its goals. This table is amplified with examples of how the different types of behaviour may be recognised.

Two popular misconceptions are revealed by looking at the work of a group in this way. The first is that ordinary members are helpless when, in fact, a great deal can be done by asking yourself 'what is missing?' and, having identified it, making a contribution that will meet this lapse. This might be getting the group to move its discussion on by doing a bit of 'clarifying' or 'summarising'; or it could be that a bit of 'gate keeping' is needed in order to bring in the shy but knowledgeable person at the end of the table. This is a very powerful tool!

The second popular misconception is that if someone is behaving negatively in ways described under 'self-oriented behaviour' it is that person's fault. If someone (maybe you) is starting to 'dominate' or 'abandon' then you know that something is wrong with the group process, that the member is not getting sufficient satisfaction out of being involved in the work and maintenance of the group. It is, of course, possible that the person is feeling tired or distracted, but on the whole there is no excuse for a meeting to be boring or unsatisfying to an essential member. Self-oriented behaviour is a symptom that the process is lacking and the balance between task and maintenance needs to be restored. It is too simple and entirely unproductive to make a personal attribution to the acting-out member. The truth of this is particularly evident when it is you who are acting out the self-oriented symptom!

There is of course a great deal more to be said about groups but in this practical pot-pourri we now turn to 'problem solving'.

Meetings and problem solving

In systems theory a problem is defined as 'the inappropriate solution imposed upon a difficulty'. I feel depressed—this is my difficulty in living (let us say that it is simply reactive to the break-up of my marriage)—so I drink: my drinking is 'the problem'. Problems in organisations are often the consequence of having to work with other people.

'Problem solving' is used here as a label to describe strategic planned thinking. Professional supervision is an example of structured thinking around a situation that needs understanding and some action or decision to be made. The structure offered here is in seven steps.

1. Collect the information—not just through collating anecdotes but in an organised way.
2. Make sense of the information by referring to past examples, theories, conceptual models and so on, so that an understanding of the situation is created.

3. Identify at least three different strategies by which to meet this situation.
4. Choose one of them.
5. Identify how you will monitor the effectiveness of the ensuing action for later reference.
6. ACT!
7. Assess the outcome.

In supervision there is a great pressure to go straight from (1) to (4) to (6). Stages (2) and (3) are needed to step out of habitual panic responses!

There are two basic approaches towards problem solving, one based on analytic thinking and the other on intuitive feeling. Both are best in their appropriate circumstances. The analytic approach is most useful when the information is available, for example when one is working out what is the best way to travel to Aberdeen: the fares and the timetables for coach, train and plane are available and the fares can be compared with travelling by car. Sometimes the information is not available—or is only available as one starts on the action. When preparing for an interview with a moody and erratic superior (or parent, or spouse), it is necessary to recognise that the careful preparation of what you will say will probably be ineffective, and will probably be entirely inappropriate. Under these circumstances the intuitive approach will be more effective, even if it is more anxiety provoking. Most people have had at least one experience of having rehearsed an interview to the extent that they are locked into that script regardless of the changed situation!

There is a wide variety of different models for problem solving. Most of them are different ways of making lists (a friend of mine says 'beat entropy, make lists!').

For an individual, when the problem solving is complete, the decision usually follows directly. In a meeting it is more complicated.

There are four main advantages to problem solving in a group:

1. It engages you in a more detailed interaction with the problem.
2. The different people can pool their different knowledge and information.
3. Errors get averaged out—and because of this people are more

willing to use their imagination, secure in the knowledge that others will be limiting any possible eccentric consequences.
4. In the security and creativity of (3) it is more likely that someone will have a 'eureka' experience of genius which will get shared around.

The disadvantages of problem solving in a group are the time it takes and that it is subject to the phenomenology of groups (see above) so well alluded to in the comment that a camel is a horse designed by a committee.

Meetings and decision making

Problem solving is at the heart of a great deal of the information processing that a meeting tackles but it is only the prelude to 'decision making'.

Problem solving is about the quality of the eventual decision, but decision making is concerned with the structure which determines the likelihood that the solution or decision will be implemented. Even the best of plans come to naught if those who have to carry them out are not committed to them.

Imagine that the principal administrator and his team have to decide between two plans, plan A and plan B. The principal favours plan A and, like everyone else; he knows that the plan he favours is the best one: he gives it a score of 100. His team favour plan B but, whilst they of course give plan B 100, the principal 'knows' that it is no more than adequate as a plan and he only gives it 70. However, the principal recognises that, if he imposes plan A (which is the best) on the team, they will only be 50% committed to implementing it and as a result, good though it is, in practice it will yield only 50% of 100 application points. He also recognises that they would be 90% committed to implementing plan B (which he knows to be inferior) but that 90% of 70 is 63 application points.

Of course, the team who thought plan B worth 100 see the application score as 90, but the principal is only concerned with his own criteria which, he sees, are better fulfilled by selecting plan B. If the figures were different, then it might be better to insist on plan A. Table 12.3 is just an example of the sorts of question that need to be asked when working in a team or an organisation.

Table 12.3

	Plan A	Plan B
Rated by principal	100	70
Commitment to implement	50%	90%
Application points	50	63

In decision making, then, it is not sufficient to arrive at the correct solution to the situation; it is also necessary to identify how to have that decision put into practice. This issue of commitment is crucial when we consider the nature of the work of the occupational therapist. There are many different structures in which decisions are made within an organisation, but the list below describes just eight of the more common structures. All things being equal, the structure and way in which a decision is made will determine the degree of involvement, responsibility and commitment to that decision of the people involved (or left out).

1. *Consensus.* Technically—and this is how we use it—this means that everyone involved supports the decision. Under the consensus structure, the decision is not ratified until everyone states their support for it.

2. *Agreement.* The decision made by agreement is one in which no-one disagrees—there may be abstentions but no voice is raised against the decision. This is sometimes known as 'nem con', for instance, the Cooperative Movement.

3. *Majority.* The decision is made when 51% of those involved support it. The constitution of an organisation, for instance, a trade union, will stipulate what sort of majority is necessary for certain sorts of decisions; the decision to strike often requires a two-thirds majority and to change the constitution may require a three-quarters majority. The two-party electoral system works on the 51% majority—but more of that later.

4. *Minority.* This is where the decision is made by a subgroup (management group, working party, sub-committee, etc.) of the decision-making body and on their behalf. This might be the executive and council of the professional body to whom will be entrusted the power to make certain decisions.

5. *Expert.* Where the decision is deferred and referred to the expert, then the group has used the 'expert structure' to make their decision. An example of this would be asking the hospital

administrative staff to allocate car parking spaces since they (presumably) are in a better position to have picked up the appropriate skills and knowledge in this area (i.e. the best places go to those who have to use their cars most frequently).

6. *Averaging*. This is where a decision is made on the basis of the replies from a questionnaire by a sort of numerical averaging. This type of decision making by averaging also occurs when a paper is circulated and you are asked for comments in the margin. The British electoral system actually works in this way when there are three or more candidates and where the elected candidate may well have only collected 34% of the votes cast.

7. *Authority with consultation*. The principal makes the first decision but he asks his colleagues for their opinions first. The staff may say all sorts of things and he listens but then makes up his own mind. It is important that the principal is not coy, talking about wanting a 'quick consensus'.

8. *Authority without consultation*. Here the principal makes up his mind, makes the decision and only later—if at all—tells the other people what was decided on their behalf. Minor day-to-day decisions are made under this structure: one hopes that the decision that these decisions may be made this way was made by a more discursive structure.

May I invite the reader to now re-read this section and check that the distinctions between structures is clear. Think of your own examples for each one.

Speaking personally, I expect all of my staff to be 100% committed to what I decide on their behalf. Bitter experience has shown me that this is insane and unrealistic: I must recognise that those decisions which require commitment also require that I allow time for the appropriate structure (Fig. 12.1), and recognise that if there is not enough support, for a decision that requires support, then the project is not viable. Similarly, it allows me to recognise those decisions which do not merit or need much time being spent on them—in this way I save the time to use it where it is needed. A colleague recently took over a very old-fashioned Elderly Persons' Home: some changes were easy and immediate—such as no longer waking all residents at 6 a.m. Other decisions, in particular the instigation of a key-worker system, took over a year to accomplish since the final decision needed the commitment that is only created by using a majority/agreement structure.

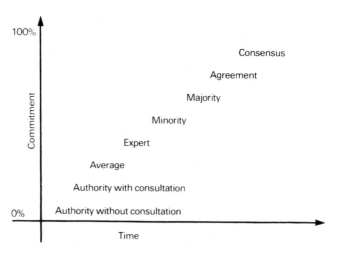

Figure 12.1 Methods of decision making related to time and commitment.

An understanding of the relationship between the decision-making structure and the commitment/time balance enables one to plan a schedule of work—and to encourage others to do the same.

It becomes clear that the meeting is not just pivotal in decision-making information processing, but that the way in which the meeting is organised, and set in the context of the rest of the members' work, determines how their work is helped or hindered by the individual and by the pattern of meetings. Before we turn to the precise duties of the chairman, let us remember the ways in which business is transacted between members of an organisation. These include the infamous 'memo', the interview with one other person, the circulation of a discussion paper (it is much easier to read a paper than to hear someone talk their way through the same material—look at the way that lecturers arrange their lectures to amplify and discuss material already read—imagine how tedious it would be if they just read out of a book to the students!).

Some organisations get stuck into the habit of long meetings which seek to do too much and consequently achieve very little. Imagine instead a meeting that is organised so that:

1. There is a brief period to catch up on any memos, reports and other bits of information best read immediately preceding the meeting.

2. There is a quarter of an hour for pairs or threes of people to quickly discuss matters that concern them only and would be tedious if discussed with the rest of the meeting as an uninvolved audience.

3. The meeting proper now starts with everyone prepared, with peripheral business complete and with members knowing that their participation will be relevant and appreciated.

4. If there is a lot of business, or if it separates into very different themes—such as administration and case discussion—then two short meetings are arranged rather than letting one impossibly demanding session be imposed upon those present.

Table 12.4 shows a structure upon which it is possible to plan decision making, general information sharing etc. and the restriction of the agenda of meetings to what is practical, necessary and viable. Try filling it in to deal with your own situation. Order the sequence of 'forums' (1, 2, 3) for the processing of each type of issue.

Chairing a meeting

The role of the chairman is crucial in a meeting. It is alarming how many people have to chair meetings who have never had the opportunity to study or learn how to do it. Some people have been lucky enough to experience good chairing from others and have learnt ways of doing it from the models provided. Other people have not had such good luck and have had rather poor models to

Table 12.4 Matching the type of decision to its appropriate level

Types of issue	Arenas or forums for the processing of information or decisions						
	Admin. officer	Snr staff meeting	Memo	Notice board	Supervision session	Staff meeting	etc.
Case							
Discussion							
Staffing							
Policy papers							
Resources							
Equipment							
Rotas							
Liaison							
Support							
etc.							
etc.							

emulate. The notes below are based on an anonymous handout I found some years ago. I am very grateful to the author and I hope that he or she would approve of the alterations and additions I have made to it over the last couple of years. You will recognise some of the concepts already described in the first part of this chapter.

It is often said that meetings comprise a bunch of the unfit, appointed by the unwilling to do the unnecessary. However, they are an intrinsic part of the work so it is necessary to make them as constructive as possible.

For the purposes of clarity and brevity this is written to emphasise the role of the chairman before, during and after meetings. This is not meant to imply that what is contained in the notes can be disregarded by those not occupying such positions. The other members need to know their roles and the process as well!

A meeting is a group and the chairman must steer the members through the inclusion stage (to create a sense of membership) and the control stage (negotiating allegiances and norms) if the discussion is to be productive. Without this, the people meeting may be more involved in working through their personal feelings and relationships than comprehending and working on the content of the meeting.

Responsibilities of a chairman

- He must earn respect.
- He must respect the views of others.
- He must control.
- He must coordinate.
- He must distinguish between opinion and fact.
- He must lead.
- He must ensure that progress is recorded.

A chairman, having accepted the role, must accept responsibility not only for the meeting but for what precedes and follows it.

Preceding the meeting

The chairman must ensure that the meeting has:

- A purpose—because this sounds obvious it is often neglected. If you haven't got a purpose you do not need a meeting.
- A secretary—provides good training for managers. Friendliness is important.

- A minute-taker—the job can be circulated. It is not a popular job but it does provide valuable training.
- An agenda—this should be as short as possible. It is better to cover a few subjects well rather than many badly.
- A date and time—if a series of meetings are planned, endeavour to fix each on a recognisable day, e.g. first Thursday of every month. Allow time prior to the meeting for up-to-date information to be gathered.
- A venue (location, accommodation, feeding)—consider the facilities required and the suitability of the room.
- Essential fittings (chairs, tables, ashtrays, paper, ventilation, etc.).
- Discussion openers and closers—prime people for these roles.
- Follow-up arrangements—action to be taken, reporting back etc.
- Winding-up arrangements—seeing people off the premises, saying goodbye, etc.

At the meeting

The agenda. The most important piece of paper at a meeting is the agenda. Like the tip of an iceberg it represents the visible portion of a large amount of otherwise unseen activity. The agenda embodies the plan of campaign which enables those responsible to achieve the objectives of the meeting. Hence, the agenda must be seen as a coherent whole, with each item contributing both to other items and the final objective. If the objective of the meeting can be summarised in about 10 lines, it will give some idea of the logical order of the items on the agenda. Some general points to be taken into account when constructing an agenda include:

- Is the early part of the agenda progressive/enthusiastic?
- The agenda can be 'timed' with the time to be allocated to urgent but unimportant items specified: with practice all items can be 'timed'.
- Can there be some items early on, on the agenda, which will be well known to most of those taking part? (This encourages participation.)
- Does it build up to a climax at the end? (An anticlimax should be avoided.)
- Do 'following' items gain strength and effect from those coming earlier?
- Are the 'controversial' items timed to coincide with the most conciliatory parts of the meeting?

- Will meal or tea breaks interfere with or help those items likely to coincide with the breaks?
- Will the inevitable latecomers or early leavers interfere with the effect of important items?

The agenda should be available before the meeting so that everyone can prepare their contribution and thoughts—thinking on one's feet is often grossly unsatisfactory.

Timing:

- The chairman needs to be in his seat at the time the meeting is due to begin. Poor timekeeping habits tend to grow. Strategies can be adopted to deal with this. Starting meetings on time even if not everybody is present tends to improve timekeeping at subsequent meetings.
- Meetings should not drag on merely to legitimate attendance. A short meeting can be favourably received. Long meetings court inattention, discomfort and irritation.
- Do keep to the stated finishing time. People who leave early assuming a meeting will drag on may be motivated to stay to the end if meetings actually finish at the time given. A stated finishing time allows people to plan other commitments—it also concentrates the mind wonderfully!

Handling personalities. It is a chairman's job to:

- inculcate a cooperative attitude
- ensure that everybody is treated with respect
- deal with one point at a time
- avoid argument early on.

Inculcate a cooperative attitude. Merely bringing people together does not mean cooperation. Cooperation means the integration of people, ideas and action in a coordinated way and this calls for listening in a positive way. The manner in which the chairman listens is contagious. Gestures, manners and refraining from other activities are all very important.

Ensure that everybody is treated with respect. Even if one disagrees there are a variety of ways in which this can be expressed, for example:

- 'That's nonsense. I don't believe a word of it. Why don't you read your papers?'

- 'The point you make might seem valid to you but I disagree, I think.'
- 'Your point is interesting and your position logical, but additional facts might lead to a different conclusion.'
- 'You have a good point, we'd like to support but . . . .'

It is important that the chairman aims to:

- understand rather than refute
- weigh the point rather than the person
- achieve progress rather than score points
- keep a neutral position.

If one has a lot to say at a meeting then probably someone else should be chairing it—a one-man show to an audience is not a meeting.

Deal with one point at a time. At any meeting there are six major roles being played, namely:

1. opinion giver
2. opinion seeker
3. fact giver
4. fact seeker
5. tester of feasibility
6. definer of problem.

Role 1 is the one adopted by most of us most of the time. Roles 5 and 6 are the ones which characterise the leaders of meetings. Being aware of this is helpful in keeping to a point and dealing with it before moving on to the next. The chairman should always summarise discussion and decisions made before moving on to the next point.

Avoid argument early on. If someone persists in opposition to a course generally supported by the others, it is often desirable for the chairman to ask the meeting if it will agree to a private discussion between the dissenter, one other interested person and himself, the decision to be reported to the next meeting. Dissension is thereby removed from the meeting and often results in a peaceful solution being found. Where a private discussion is not feasible, the disagreement and dissenter should be respected and the issue closed, moving on to the next point before the proceedings are poisoned!

After the meeting. The follow-up is the test of a good meeting. Points to be watched for include:

1. Each decision to be implemented should be associated with a time and date of completion. A margin on the right of a page can be used for this recording.

2. Individuals responsible for implementing decisions should have their names clearly recorded in the minutes together with the name of the person to whom completion is to be reported.

3. The minutes should be concise—not more than two pages—and circulated as quickly as possible. They could be typed and copied whilst the meeting is wound up.

4. Progress should be reported at the next meeting; this is important if people are to feel accountable.

At this point one reaches full circle. What follows one meeting precedes the next. In this context the significance of asking questions in the right way becomes important. For written questions the following points are useful:

- Put a heading on the paper which catches the eye and interest of the person receiving it. This not only helps in achieving action, but it helps to identify the paper and assists filing.
- Be concise.
- Seek commitment. For 'no' answers ask for specific reasons.
- Ask for confirmation of set targets and dates.
- Attempt to make the question as meaningful to the person being asked for information as to the person seeking information.
- If a question is directed at a number of people, they should all see the replies.
- For circulated questions/information, include a circulation list.
- Put a reminder in your diary when such follow-up is to be initiated.

The chairman will find the execution of these duties slightly eased if he bears the previous sections in mind. For instance, in chairing discussion, it is useful to be able to follow the problem-solving structure of organising discussion:

1. Collect information and describe the problem, and only then
2. Make sense of it, and only after that
3. Let the discussion move on to considering solutions and strategies.

You may wish to photocopy this section and give it to the person who chairs some of your own meetings. This is, of course, illegal and infringes the copyright rules, so lend him or her the book.

CONFLICT AND NEGOTIATION
Winning and losing

On occasions the occupational therapist is offered the chance to be in conflict with someone else. You can always decline this invitation if it does not suit you. There is no point in entering a conflict or fight if you are going to lose. Of course, you may be prepared to lose in one area if there is a trade-off somewhere else, or there will be a definite benefit in the longer term. Indeed, on matters of principle you will fight because not to fight would be truly to lose, whereas to lose that particular battle is, in fact, to win.

Let us, then, look at a framework for conflict and at strategies of negotiation. Galvin Whitaker says that one should always be able to answer two questions before proceeding. The first is: 'What is the price of winning?' You may recall that Lt Calley, charged with the massacre of Vietnamese villagers, answered in his defence, 'in order to save the village we had to destroy it'. There are many times when the price of winning is too great and under those circumstances it is better not to fight.

The second question is: 'Whose will will prevail?' If the odds are against you, do not fight! Wait until the odds are in your favour. The more important the issue the more important it is to act with circumspection, discretion and success.

There is a famous parable called 'Prisoner's dilemma' that is told to illustrate the problems of conflict. Jake and Bill meet up one day and decide to rob a bank. They are exceedingly good at robbing banks. They do the job and get back home and into bed by 3 a.m. Suddenly there is a knock on the door; 'Open up in the name of the Law' comes the demand. To cut a longer story short, they are taken down to the police station, put in separate cells, and after an hour or so, the Inspector visits each of them in turn and says, 'We know you did it, lad. Now do us a good turn and do yourself a favour. Turn Queen's evidence on the other fellow and we'll drop the charge against you.'

The dilemma is as follows: if they both deny the charge, they both get off because the police cannot make the charge stick. If one of them grasses on the other whilst that other is still denying the charge, then the grass gets off and the other one takes the full rap—and, further, the grass does not have to share the stashed loot with him. But, if they both grass, then there is evidence on them both and they both go down, although not for as long as if either took the sole rap. Figure 12.2 shows the dilemma.

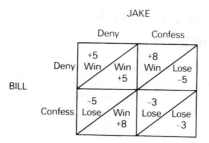

Figure 12.2 The win–lose game in negotiation.

What would you do? If you can be absolutely sure of Jake, then, as Bill, you deny the charge. Or, if you are sure that he will not grass on you, then you can grass on him and get his share of the haul. But if you deny the charge and he grasses on you, then he gets your share. It is a pretty little game to play over 10 rounds because once one person—say Bill—breaks faith, then Jake is likely to grass back on him, because that way he will lose less by doing so than he would lose through trusting Bill. Once one person starts playing about and acting greedy it is very difficult to regain the situation in the top left-hand box of Figure 12.2— and that is a chronic problem, even if the people concerned are colleagues involved in, for example, occupational therapy.

We have, then, the Win/Win box, the Win/Lose boxes and the Lose/Lose box. As long as both occupational therapist and charge nurse are working together on a Win/Win strategy there is a basic positive pay-off for them both, they make five points each every day and take home 25 units of well-being and satisfaction at the end of the week. We can, of course, imagine a situation where they distrust each other and expect the worst of each other and play safe in the Lose/Lose box in which the most that they can lose is three points—and they just might make an eight now and again. At the end of the week this war of attrition will have taken its toll in a quiet and persistent fashion, but the most they can lose is $3 \times 5 = 15$ and that is certainly better than having risked the Win/Lose box and lost each day, thus losing a total of $5 \times 5 = 25$ points. In the first instance they were choosing a strategy whereby to maximise their gains: in the second it was the strategy of minimising their losses.

The problem, of course, is what to do when you are working with someone in order to maximise your gains and suddenly he or she lands you a minus five. Suddenly you are let down by your colleague and you need to work out what to do. What we know is that there is an inexorable logic which pulls interdependent outcomes such as this one through the Win/Lose box. Having been let down once, why not a second time? Should I punish my colleague and get my own back when next I have a chance? If I say nothing, does that give the impression that I can be pushed around?

Fortunately, occupational therapists do not work in separate cells and so there is the possibility of discussing the matter with your colleague who might have made a mistake, might also have got a minus five from the interaction since a third party had let her down; or she might indeed have been trying to pull a fast one on you and you need to show her that this road leads to both of you faring worse in the long term, even if in the short term there is some advantage for her. Everyone always lets someone down every day—it is important to devise a structure and understanding that keeps you off the slippery Win/Lose slope that leads to Lose/Lose. You might like to take a moment and think about the dilemma of the situation in which you 'can win the battle at the cost of the war'.

You might like now to consider how you would recognise a situation in which your 'colleague' was so mean and wretched that you have to work a 'minimise your losses strategy'. (Consider also that life is too short to waste in a Lose/Lose game—when I talk with people who have left unsatisfactory workplaces, they usually say, 'I should have left a couple of years earlier'; learn from their experience; if the writing is on the wall, recognise it before you get exhausted!)

Figure 12.3 describes the two basic dimensions of a conflict situation. The mode of resolution of the conflict depends upon:

1. the assertiveness of each party in pursuing his or her own goals; and
2. how cooperative each person is in pursuing the goals of the other party.

The final mode of resolution depends upon where each person is on each of these two dimensions. Let us first consider Sue: if she is assertive and cooperative, then she is likely to be offering a collaborative solution; if she is neither concerned about her own goals nor Janet's goals, then she will offer to avoid any conflict; if she is concerned about her own goals but not about Janet's, then she will offer a competition between the two of them...and so on. Janet's position is similarly identified. The outcome of their conflict will be a product of how their stances and invitation to each other mesh together. The style Janet adopts interacts with the style Sue favours and the actual way in which they deal with this situation is a product of the two styles in interaction. You might like to consider some of the issues that feature in a couple of your relationships and work out how this model fits what actually happens. Remember that, if this is your relationship with a colleague, then the outcome affects your patients, not just yourselves; and recognise how concern for the other person's goals makes it more likely that—in the long term as in the prisoner's dilemma—individually and collectively you will benefit!

Strategies

There are a number of different ways in which a conflict of interests can be conducted. It is very important to be able to determine which is the structure of resolution that is most appropriate to the particular situation.

Conversion

My response to our conflict of interests—or beliefs—is to attempt to convert you to my way of thinking. I attempt this through force of argument, personality or threat. There are certainly times

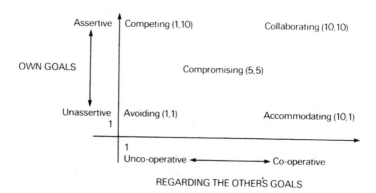

Figure 12.3 Gains in different styles of negotiation (Blake & Mouton 1964).

when this is effective and appropriate but it can also serve to make the conflict worse and generate a lot of bad feeling that could be very unfortunate in the long run.

Joint problem solving

This is where we both recognise the situation we are in and set about working together on a joint goal that will permit both of us to gain our own goals en route. We put our cards on the table and try to understand each other's position and, working together, hope to find a resolution in which we both get all that we want. For instance, instead of competing for certain limited resources, we decide to work together to increase the total amount of resources so that we can then split them up, each getting as much, or more, than would have been the case had we disputed for them. However, if your protagonist does not want to work with you in this way, you may have put yourself at a grave disadvantage and may well end up merely giving in stages! A second problem is that, if it is not possible (in the above example) to get extra resources or to get a consensus between the various parties, the conflict just goes on in an inconclusive way causing much delay and frustration.

Negotiation

This is a more expensive structure than problem solving since it involves the trading of concessions. In problem solving you hope to make no concessions but in negotiation the exchange of concessions is the essential component of the conversations towards resolution. Many people feel nervous about negotiation—they fear being out-manoeuvred and taken advantage of by the other person and therefore refuse to negotiate. Where problem solving is inappropriate, conversion is ineffective and negotiation is not available, then all that is left is a stand-off with neither person getting even a bit of what he or she needs or wants.

There is a structure of four phases in negotiation and if you are aware of the sequence of phases and how to manage each one it is likely that you will be able to negotiate a way that brings satisfaction to you—and also to the other person. Remember, if the other person feels that he has been taken advantage of, he will not work well with you.

The stages are as follows:

1. *Prepare.* Define your objective and work out your preferred and your minimum positions so that you can identify what concessions you are prepared to exchange. Work out what information you need and get it—especially about what the others want of the deal. Then prepare yourself a simple strategy for the following:

2. *Argue and discuss.* State your opening (and realistic) position and listen to his. Test out assumptions you have made and exchange information and learn what is important to him as well as what is important to you, and signal your interest in continuing to talk. 'There are our standard charges . . .,' 'that would be very difficult to agree to . . .' and '. . . as things stand' are all ways of signalling that the situation is open to further negotiation!

3. *Propose.* You next move to making suggestions in order to advance the negotiation. 'What if . . .', '. . . could consider . . . may be'. Do not interrupt, just listen to the suggestions, question them, summarise them and offer counter-proposals until you both feel you have an idea of the width and limits of the other person's thoughts. Then construct a 'package'—re-present the original proposal in a different form in the light of what you have learnt in the foregoing discussions.

4. *Bargain.* This only happens after the preparatory phases have been explored. This is where, having got a good idea of what is important to the other person, you can start to trade concessions. The formula is clear; if you will do X, then I will concede Y; state the condition before the offer and never concede anything without something being given in return. Bit by bit the two parties move closer together (or one party realises that no realistic and satisfactory deal is possible) and eventually one person moves to the 'close' by trading a final concession for a deal: 'If you will throw in Z then we have a deal'.

And finally you both agree what was agreed, summarise and record the resolution so that when you need to re-negotiate it some time in the future you both know where you are starting from.

Do not rush negotiations. Take your time and take pauses to think. Do not get to the bargaining stage too soon or you may well find that you miss opportunities to create a deal that satisfies both yourself and the other person—with whom you probably have to work for the next few years!

To review this immediate passage, there are several different structures for organising the resolution of conflicts and differences of interest. It is important to identify which structure is appropriate for any situation so that the most fruitful resolution can be found. There is no special merit in any one structure but there is a grave danger of finding yourself doing one approach when the other person is using a different one.

The key note in this section has been that it is legitimate and necessary to recognise that the handling of conflict and the selection of strategies for negotiation are professional tasks and need to be thought about and planned like all other interventions in one's professional life. If you count up the percentage of the working week spent in such negotiations, and if you consider how these bits balance those that are more directly related to your clients, then you realise that you get a third of your money for exercising these particular skills!

But, before we move to the final section, a very useful quotation taken from 'Illuminatus' by Shea & Wilson (1977) (for redundant read 'rigid'):

People exist on a spectrum from the most redundant to the most flexible. The latter, unless they are thoroughly trained in psychodynamics, are always at a disadvantage to the former in social interactions. The redundant do not change their script; the flexible continually keep changing, trying to find a way of relating constructively. Eventually the flexible ones find the 'power' gambit, and communication, of a sort, is possible. They are now on the set created by the redundant person, and they act out his or her script.

The steady exponential growth of bureaucracy is not due to Parkinson's Law alone. The State, by making itself even more redundant, incorporates more people into its set and forces them to follow its script.

Power, responsibility and information

There is a constant conservative tendency of people and organisations to attribute the cause of someone's behaviour to his personality. Some years back I ran some research on this subject and had my suspicions confirmed: when asked why someone does a thing—such as shout at a dog—people replied that the man shouted at the dog because he was that sort of a man. When asked why they might shout at a dog they attributed the cause to external factors—such as the dog's behaviour. The world is a simpler, more manageable place if we just see the cause for a person's behaviour in his or her 'personality', even though we know perfectly well that if we were to do it—or people we know well were to do it—we would look beyond the personality for an explanation of behaviour.

When there is a difficulty or failing in part of an organisation, the organisation will tend to attribute the cause to the personalities of the people involved or responsible. However, if you speak with the persons involved, it is often the case that they can identify other reasons—such as a poor line of communication, lack of secretarial assistance, a qualitative change in the severity of the handicap of the client group, etc.—which have caused the pressure and the failure. The organisation will attribute the cause to the 'personalities' of those involved since it can follow that diagnosis with the prescription that they should change. Were the organisation to realise that it was a structurally induced failure, then the organisation would have to change—which is less readily perceived by those in a position to effect it. You can probably identify certain posts in your organisation in which, whoever occupies them, the work is impaired and the occupants blamed. Such posts have a high turnover but each occupant gets blamed in turn for a structurally induced handicap. Avoid such a post.

You will remember from the discussion of groups that the individual who is expressing boredom and dissatisfaction can either be seen as a disruptive personality or as the member expressing the group's malfunction. It is the same thing.

Dorothy and Galvin Whitaker, respectively Professor of Social Work at York University and Reader in Management Studies at Leeds University, recommend the following diagnostic structure for examining the performance of a task in an organisation. It is derived from a psychotherapeutic model of effectiveness.

$$\text{Task} \rightarrow (\text{Power} \equiv \text{Responsibility} \equiv \text{Information}) \times \text{Competence}$$

Thus, in considering the work performed by a staff member, first it is necessary to identify the specific tasks that he or she performs and to check whether this information has been made available to the worker. It is common to find people employed on one job description and yet expected to fulfil a different one.

The effectiveness of the work performance to this task is dependent upon four further factors. The natural conservatism of organisations leads one to first enquire after the competence of the staff member and, as suggested earlier, to ask no further. However, this present model obliges one to recognise the following dynamic as being the modifier of such competence in practice.

The amount of responsibility allocated to a worker must be balanced by a commensurate amount of power and also a commensurate amount of information (information about both his own role and duties and also the wider context of the purpose of the work). Responsibility and power without sufficient information will make the best of workers a menace to his colleagues: the best truck driver in a powerful vehicle for which he is responsible is dangerous if his windscreen is whitewashed. Another example often quoted is of certain senior administrators who have undoubted qualities, responsibility and power, but who do not actually know what is happening in certain portions—operational portions— of their organisation. Should they be sacked for incompetence or do we look to see how to supply the necessary information? We will then know to sack them if they cannot manage their jobs.

Responsibility and information without commensurate level of power renders the worker helpless. Either the accountability/ responsibility must be reduced or the discretion and power must be increased because until that time it is unlikely that this helpless worker will be able to perform the tasks adequately.

Power and information without responsibility is another imbalanced and destructive situation, although not as crippling as the previous examples. This can occur when a receptionist achieves influence on the informal communication network and, as usual, knows more of what is happening around an organisation than anyone else: if she gets bored or annoyed she is in a position to guide the affairs without being responsible for the outcome.

We look at the occupational therapist's performance and we ask about the external situational factors such as how clearly the task is defined, how the power, information and responsibility factors are balanced before we presume to assess her competence. The approach also allows us to diagnose an organisation by taking different sections and different posts within it and asking these questions, rather than glibly saying that of course the occupational therapy department is a mess, look at the head occupational therapist, or 'no wonder that psychiatrist is a disaster to his patients, look at the bumbling arrogant way the visits are arranged'. Instead, you ask the questions and refrain from making personal attributions until it is appropriate; if it is appropriate.

You will find this equation invaluable; commit it to your memory, use if often and look for the situational factors before you start criticising others. Maybe others will do this for you, too. Maybe.

REFERENCES

Blake R R, Mouton J S 1964 The managerial grid. Gulf Publishing, Texas
Schutz W C 1958 FIRO: a 3D theory of interpersonal behaviour. Rinehart, New York
Shea R, Wilson A 1977 The golden apple. Sphere, New York

Index